Creating Practice-based Evidence

Library of Congress Cataloguing in Publication Data
British Library Cataloguing in Publication Data
A catalogue record for this book is available from the British Library
Cover design: Jim Wilkie
Project management, typesetting and design: J&R Publishing Services Ltd, Guildford, Surrey, UK; www.jr-publishingservices.co.uk

Printed and bound by CPI Group (UK) Ltd, Croydon, CR0 4YY

Creating Practice-based Evidence

A guide for SLTs

Corinne Dobinson and Yvonne Wren
(Editors)

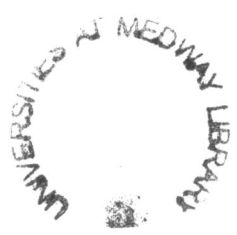

J&R Press Ltd

Contents

List of figures

List of tables

Foreword

Most of us endeavour to provide evidence-based care but in many cases this is difficult as it is hard to translate research into clinical practice and, less obviously, it is demanding to relate clinical practice to research. Trying to bring these two worlds together is vitally important at this time when our interventions are being more closely inspected by patients, carers, other professionals and those who purchase our services. Thus, it is essential to bridge the clinician–researcher divide if patient care is to become explicitly cost effective. This requires the right questions to be asked, the correct methods to be chosen, appropriate analysis and effective dissemination.

The research and clinical cultures are different and have different incentives, regimes and languages. Multiculturalism requires respect and knowledge of the semantics of the language as well as the taboos! This book can be viewed as an anthropological study, allowing explorers to venture into new worlds and appreciate the opportunities afforded by such exposure and experience. It provides a 'Lonely Planet Guide' to both the newcomer to this world as well as the more experienced traveller, allowing the reader to select the areas which will be of most importance and relevance at any one time.

The book will also give confidence to those wishing to venture into new territory by providing easily-understood information on which to base research and evaluation of their own practice. This will add to or replace the clinical anecdote with explicit and reproducible evidence. If all speech and language therapists were able to collect robust information on each of their clients and how they respond to different interventions, we would then be in a different world!

Pam Enderby
Professor of Community Rehabilitation
Sheffield, UK
July 2012

Preface

The motivation for writing a book on creating practice-based evidence arose as a consequence of the editors' experiences in both research and clinical roles. We both returned to clinical practice after being engaged solely in speech and language therapy research while completing our PhDs. Working once again as clinicians under the constraints of the NHS, and the daily challenges this presents, was a stark reminder of the difficulties faced by clinicians in using the evidence base and in making contributions towards it. SLTs are continually being asked to support their clinical practice and service development with evidence, yet many may feel too inexperienced or find they have insufficient time to gather evidence from the literature or, more specifically, from their own clinical work. Moreover, without a local research culture to support such activities, this is even more challenging. Our own experience was that there seemed to be a research–clinical divide; leaving research and evidence-gathering mainly to the academic and clinical service delivery to the clinician.

Having a foot in both camps, so to speak, we recognized that clinicians' queries, and sometimes uncertainties, about everyday clinical practice are a rich resource. These form the foundations of valuable evidence-gathering, since they originate from the interface of service provision and service user; the real world of SLT with all its challenges. We therefore felt that a book on how to create evidence from everyday clinical practice could offer clinicians who have little research experience the opportunity to begin to contribute to the evidence base, right from the clinic room; ultimately, by combining clinical practice and research activities.

The Royal College of Speech and Language Therapists (RCSLT) began to develop its research strategy around the same time that we had the idea for the book. The strategy aims to develop and support a research culture across the profession, and to provide a framework and guidance to facilitate this process.

We hope that you find the following chapters not only useful as a guide in gathering evidence in the workplace, but also a source of encouragement as you engage in that process.

Corinne Dobinson and Yvonne Wren
Bristol, July 2012

Acknowledgements

We would like to thank Sue Roulstone and Rosemarie Hayhow for their assistance in the early stages of developing this book. We would also like to express our thanks to Sophie Slade, Hayley Wilmott-Taylor, Emily Highfield, Diana Benton and Rebecca Coad who gave valuable feedback on the first drafts of the chapters. Finally, we are grateful to Rachael Wilkie from J&R Press for her advice and support throughout the editing of this book.

About the authors

Wendy Best

Wendy Best is a Research Speech and Language Therapist, and Professor of Communication Science and Language Therapy at UCL. She started her career working with children in community clinics and then worked with adults with aphasia. While working in universities she has maintained strong clinical links by visiting students on placement, working on research projects with colleagues employed in the NHS and, most recently, in a part-time role in clinical supervision for therapists working with children with language needs. She directs the Centre for Speech and Language Intervention Research which promotes links between research and practice.

Steven Bloch

Steven qualified from Birmingham Polytechnic as a Speech and Language Therapist in 1991. His clinical and research interests have focused on everyday conversations between people with progressive neurological diseases and their families. As a clinician with a wide range of community intervention experiences he has always been keen to promote the importance of everyday life in clinical work. Following his PhD in 2006, Steven has worked at University College London. He is currently a National Institute for Health Research Fellow and an associate editor of the *International Journal of Language and Communication Disorders*.

Jan Broomfield

Dr Jan Broomfield worked as an NHS Speech and Language Therapist for 30 years until February 2011 when she moved into independent practice. She works with children, lectures at Newcastle University and runs EBP workshops for clinicians. Jan's PhD, completed in 2003, involved a clinical effectiveness RCT of 730 children with primary communication impairment; findings have been widely published. Jan then became a Consultant SLT, specialising in child speech disorder, continuing to be involved in research and working with the RCSLT, leading the development of their Developmental Verbal Dyspraxia Policy Statement and being Research and Development Councillor between 2009 and 2012.

Corinne Dobinson

Corinne Dobinson is a Speech and Language Therapist who has over 30 years of clinical experience. She completed her MSc while specialising in voice disorders, before developing a further specialism in adult acquired neurology. She completed her PhD in 2007, developing and evaluating dysarthria software for home practice. She then returned to clinical practice, working with adults who have communication difficulties associated with neurological problems and stroke. In addition to her clinical work, Corinne is research active and has a specialist role to support the SLT service in matters of research and to promote this in the workplace.

Rosemarie Hayhow

Rosemarie Hayhow, Speech and Language Therapist, has been fortunate to work with children and adults who stammer for nearly 40 years. Throughout this time her clinical, educational and research work have been fuelled by the desire to gain a better understanding of stammering and the related therapeutic approaches. The challenge of continuing to develop therapy skills while gaining a deeper understanding of treatment mechanisms and their applicability has ensured a stimulating career. Curiosity about what we do, why we do it and whether we could be more effective leads to uncertainty but can also stimulate research and so foster continued development.

Chris Markham

Chris Markham began working as a Generalist Speech and Language Therapist in hospital rehabilitation and community clinics before specialising in Special Educational Needs. His interest in research was inspired by the communication needs he encountered on a daily basis. Chris carried out his MSc project alongside his clinical role, which cultivated a greater passion for evidence-based practice. His Doctoral Fellowship involved designing and validating a quality of life measure for children who have communication needs. Chris is currently Course Leader for the Foundation Degree in speech, language and communication sciences at Portsmouth University where he continues his research.

Nick Miller

Nick Miller is a Speech and Language Therapist by background with many years' clinical experience in paediatric and acquired neurological posts. He is currently lecturer, clinician and researcher in communication disorders at the University of Newcastle, UK. His chief research interest lies in motor speech disorders (he is national advisor to the Royal College of Speech and Language Therapists), with communication changes in cerebral palsy and in Parkinson's a central focus. His work encompasses all aspects of motor speech disorders, from the underlying nature of communication impairment in neurological conditions through to the psychosocial impact on the person and their family.

Hazel Roddam

Hazel worked as a clinical SLT for 25 years in a range of health and education settings. She worked predominantly in the field of learning difficulties and physical disabilities, with a particular interest in introducing AAC systems to young children with cerebral palsy. Hazel's research over the past 10 years has focused on perceptions of evidence-based practice and the influences on therapists' clinical decision-making. Hazel took up her post at the University of Central Lancashire in 2006 and has worked to build increased collaborative links with local clinicians, to focus on applied research on clinical topics and workforce issues.

Sue Roulstone

Sue Roulstone is Underwood Trust Professor of Language and Communication Impairment at the University of the West of England, Bristol. Sue's clinical speciality is with preschool children and she was head of department for Bristol's children's speech and language therapy before taking up her current role as a Director of the Bristol Speech & Language Therapy Research Unit. Her research interests include child and family perspectives, professional judgement and evaluation of speech and language therapy. Sue was Chair of the Royal College of Speech and Language Therapists from 2004–2006.

Helen Stringer

Helen Stringer is a dual qualified Speech and Language Therapist and teacher specialising in developmental communication disorders. Helen completed her PhD, 'Children and adolescents with language and behaviour disorders', while practising as an SLT in the NHS. She currently works at Newcastle University researching into interventions for children with complex speech disorders and co-occurring language and behaviour disorders. Helen is the Director of the MSc in Evidence Based Practice in Communication Disorders and a founding member of the North East SLT Research Collaboration, both aimed at encouraging and supporting SLTs to research their clinical practice.

Yvonne Wren

Yvonne Wren worked as a clinician covering both adult and child caseloads for ten years before embarking on a research career. Her research activity has focused on speech development as well as understanding the range and delivery of interventions used with children. Yvonne's PhD investigated the use of software in intervention for children's speech disorders and this led to the development of the Phoneme Factory software series. She has been co-applicant and lead applicant on a number of small- and large-scale studies but has sought to maintain her skills as a clinician through ongoing assessments and intervention to ensure her research is grounded in everyday practice.

Part I Getting started

1 Practice-based evidence: What is it and why do we need it?

Corinne Dobinson and Yvonne Wren

Learning outcomes

By the end of this chapter, you will know and understand:

- What is meant by practice-based evidence
- What constitutes evidence
- The drivers for SLT research
- The aim of the book and how to use it
- The framework for NHS research
- Where small-scale research fits in

Introduction

We have all had those times in our working lives when our intuition tells us that a different approach might work better for our client. This could be an alternative method of working taken from existing approaches or, indeed, something developed on the spot, based on reasoning from our knowledge and experience. It's what makes our job as Speech and Language Therapists (SLTs) both creative and rational. Alternatively, through our clinical practice, we might feel unconvinced that a particular approach works very well, or we might find it is difficult to deliver. At other times, we might feel that increasing numbers of clients with a particular type of problem have been walking through our door during the past few years or, alternatively, that referral rates are dropping. These insightful hunches are the forerunner of good clinical research questions and practising SLTs are ideally placed to generate them.

There are a number of reasons, though, why we might not take these ideas further and develop them into research questions, including lack of time, lack of confidence in our skills as a researcher, or maybe an opinion that clinical research is best left to the academics. One can certainly feel overawed by the achievements of some researchers and the research world can feel exclusive to some clinicians. However, if we embed gathering evidence within our own clinical activity our skills will develop, and it can help us to answer some of these intuitive queries more confidently.

The term *practice-based evidence* succinctly defines gathering evidence during the course of everyday clinical activity. This means generating a question that is based on a concern, query or hunch about your current way of working and approaching that question methodically in order to answer it as best you can within the resources available to you. By incorporating such activities into everyday work, you can, with the right support, build confidence in gathering evidence and finding answers to the questions that you want to ask. Indeed, ultimately you might collaborate with others to build up a rich source of data that can inform clinical practice and support your decision-making. Key to this will be to know what support and resources you need and where to find them. This book aims to be one such resource.

The drive for evidence-based practice

What is evidence?

Evidence is generally thought of as proof which supports a claim or belief. In health service delivery, this might be interpreted as proof that an intervention works, proof that a proportion of our caseload has a specific problem or proof that an intervention is acceptable (or not). Increasingly, we are expected to provide such proof in our clinical workplace to support our services; this could be to justify the use of a particular approach or intervention, to provide relevant information for commissioning purposes or to make sure we are working efficiently.

Drivers for SLT research and the RCSLT research strategy

In 2009, The Royal College of Speech and Language Therapists (RCSLT) developed and published its research strategy in response to drivers for evidence-based practice. The aim of the publication is to support and guide SLTs in matters of research (Royal College of Speech and Language Therapists, 2009). Briefly, the objectives of the SLT research strategy are to use, contribute to and support the development of the evidence base in order to: achieve the best outcomes for service users and RCSLT members; meet the demands of commissioners, service planners and purchasers who want evidence-based services; support the NHS requirement of delivering evidence-based services; and inform national policy decisions. It aims to do this by building the research capacity in the profession so that SLTs can use and contribute to the evidence base.

The move towards supporting a research culture in the profession is clearly stated. All SLTs have a research component to their job descriptions reflecting the level of engagement for their particular banding. Guidance documents can be found on the RCSLT website which state what research activities these might include.

Implementation of the research strategy is being achieved by giving it a prominent place in RCSLT conferences and developing the role of Special Interest Groups in this respect so they can support it. There have also been a number of excellent articles published in *Bulletin* and other publications to assist SLTs to use the evidence base to support clinical decision-making. In addition, RCSLT has become a member of the Allied Health Professions Research Network. This serves to build the research capacity and capability of the allied health professions, to support the implementation of the evidence into clinical practice and to increase access to the knowledge base; details can be found on the RCSLT website.

Types of evidence

When we think of evidence-based practice (EBP), we tend to think of research evidence, but there are other sorts of evidence you could be interested in gathering in your clinic. Increasingly in clinical practice, the triad of evidence-based practice is being used; evidence relating to systematic research is complemented by evidence from clinical expertise and evidence of patient or client preferences (Dollaghan, 2007). Evidence can also be considered more broadly to include service evaluation and audit as well as empirical research – but what's the difference?

Research generates *new* knowledge about causes, relationships, views and perceptions; service evaluation looks at the *standard* that is achieved by a service; audit measures service outcomes and compares these with a pre-determined standard, to see if current service delivery is meeting those standards. It is important to know the difference between these types of evidence, even though it can be a grey area in places, as the type of evidence will determine whether or not you need certain approvals to carry out a project. You may therefore feel you need to seek advice about where your project sits within these types.

The aim of this book

The idea behind this book, and that of the people who have contributed to it, is to bridge the gap between clinical practice and active research. By guiding and encouraging clinicians to use their everyday practice as a platform for gathering evidence, it aims to help SLTs cultivate and develop research thinking and to make research more inclusive. Ultimately, it aims to help SLTs find solutions to the questions that arise in the clinical context and to have increased confidence when working clinically or meeting commissioners of our services. We have therefore aimed, all the way through the book, to be sympathetic to the clinician with an understanding of the constraints within which they operate.

When starting out with our idea, we wanted to feel confident that the book would address real clinical issues that SLTs are concerned about and want to investigate. We therefore asked a number of clinicians who work with different client groups to identify the types of clinical questions they would like answers to. In addition, we asked what their concerns were in clinical practice and what issues they felt unsure about. We also asked them to consider which research question they would like to address if the necessary resources were available to them. The themes of these questions form the chapter headings and subject matter of the book.

As the main focus of this book is to help SLTs get started in evidence gathering, small-scale research is particularly relevant, but we also provide guidance for those wishing to take things to the next level. We have therefore included information that is helpful in guiding smaller- and larger-scale investigations using a range of research methods. Whilst we cannot provide an exhaustive list of methods or analyses that can be used in gathering evidence, we have provided information on some approaches to data collection that fit with the types of clinical questions you might want to ask. Importantly, we have tried to take into account the constraints on resources and suggested how you might gather evidence within these limitations. We have also given further reading recommendations to guide readers to more detailed literature and, where possible, have provided other useful resources.

Evidence gathering has its own terminology and style and can alienate those who are not familiar with it. With that in mind, our aim was to make the tone of the book friendly and accessible, while helping the reader to begin to feel comfortable with research terminology; we have therefore defined terms that might be new and included a glossary. In addition, we have included learning outcomes at the beginning of each chapter and summaries at the end to draw the main points together.

It was important to us that our contributors would be able to empathise with the clinician. Although our contributing authors are experienced in carrying out research, all of them have SLT clinical backgrounds. At some point, they all took their first steps in gathering evidence more formally.

Layout of the book

As you will see, we have divided the book into three sections. Part I addresses general issues around gathering evidence, Part II gives guidance on answering the types of question clinicians might want to ask, and Part III provides advice that fits in with the final stages of evidence gathering and when considering moving on to another stage in research activity.

Part I begins with our own introductory chapter. Here we provide an overview of the drivers for practice-based evidence and the frameworks for evaluating complex interventions; showing how small-scale research fits into these. We also provide background information about how research is supported within the NHS. In Chapter 2, Sue Roulstone and Rosemarie Hayhow explain the process of gathering evidence. Specifically, they illustrate the stages involved and provide a useful flowchart of these for easy reference. Helen Stringer, in Chapter 3, addresses issues around the practicalities of conducting research; she provides valuable advice about where to find support and tips on how to make the process described in Chapter 2 progress smoothly.

Part II focuses on the 'nitty gritty' of addressing clinical questions which are of interest to SLTs and which form the basis for research. A question we commonly ask is whether or not our intervention changes a client's impairment. This is the subject of Chapter 4, where Corinne Dobinson and Nick Miller assist the clinician–researcher in answering this question. They ask us to think carefully about defining our terms and procedures and to ensure we have controlled for bias as much as is possible, and suggest suitable approaches a clinician–researcher might use.

For almost all of our clients the aim of making changes in impairment is to improve life opportunities; in Chapter 5, Chris Markham assists us in investigating the impact of our intervention on quality of life. He addresses issues around the definition and measurement of quality of life and clients' levels of activity and participation.

In evaluating our intervention or services it is important to have knowledge of the views and experiences of clients and others. Steven Bloch and Wendy Best help us with this in Chapter 6. They illustrate some of the difficulties that can be involved in trying to get an accurate picture of the perspectives of others whilst suggesting practical ways to achieve this.

We are often engaged in training activities, imparting knowledge and advice to others who might be working with our clients. In Chapter 7, Yvonne Wren gives guidance on evaluating this not only in terms of how our training impacts on the trainee but also, importantly, the client group.

Sometimes, we need to know how many clients we see who fall into a specific group; this could relate to type of communication problem, age group, or other demographic data. In Chapter 8, Jan Broomfield gives us guidance on how to use existing data sources to gather and analyze such information and also how to gather other important data on caseloads such as outcomes.

In Part III, topics are addressed which are particularly useful when evidence-gathering has finished, but that we need to consider as we go along. Rosemarie Hayhow, in Chapter 9, highlights the importance of disseminating findings. She gives advice and tips on how to present our results to different audiences using different media. In Chapter 10, Hazel Roddam guides those of us who would like to move on in personal development, should we get the research bug. She provides guidance on applying for higher degrees and where to get funding to take our research forward. In Chapter 11, we summarize the key points with the intention of leaving the reader ready and equipped to start gathering evidence. The book is a reference guide which can be dipped into or used in a more structured way depending on your particular needs. The next section makes suggestions on how you might like to use it.

How to use this book

If you are new to research and want to gain an overview of the processes involved and mandatory requirements, Part I provides you with the information you need to develop an initial idea and turn it into a research proposal. Chapter 1 will provide you with background information about how the NHS is supported to carry out research and where small-scale research fits into models for evaluating complex interventions. Chapter 2 will take you through the processes step by step, while Chapter 3 will help with the detail of achieving each of the steps.

Once you have an overview of the processes involved and the practical issues you need to consider, identify which of the chapters in Part II is most relevant to the broader question you want to answer. These chapters will help you build on your reading from Chapters 2 and 3 by addressing specific issues in relation to your particular question, and your research plan will become increasingly detailed and refined. This will give you the best opportunity of answering your question and, if necessary, securing funds to help you do this.

Part III needs to be considered alongside the chapters in Parts I and II. Whatever research or evaluation activity you carry out, you will need to write an account of your work. This could be anything from a report for commissioners of clinical services, the funders of the research or the individual who requested the information, to a formal paper for submission for peer review publication. As many experienced researchers will testify, it is best to avoid leaving the writing up until the end of the project. A much more efficient and less stressful approach is to write as you progress through your research plan. For this reason, it would be helpful to read Chapter 9 as you develop your research plan and build time into your proposal for writing. In addition, whilst you might want to leave plans to apply for research degrees or further funding until you have finished this first project, bear in mind that funding bodies require several months to consider an application before confirming whether or not the monies will be awarded. You might therefore find the guidance in Chapter 10 useful in the early stages of your research as you consider what the next steps might be when you have completed your current project.

Frameworks for clinical outcome research

When researching 'in the lab', so to speak, conditions are controlled to the extent where it is possible to isolate, with reasonable reliability, the factors that determine, or have relationships with, other factors. However, there are many facets to communication and swallowing interventions that make them complex, meaning there are a number of factors that can influence an outcome.

One example of a complex intervention, from many within the field of speech and language therapy, is intervention for developmental speech impairment. Promoting change in a child's speech sound system is not a simple task. In common with other areas of speech and language therapy, it cannot be achieved through the administration of a single procedure. Factors that could affect the outcome of intervention include: number and frequency of therapy sessions; use of parents or teachers or others as agents of therapy; location of therapy sessions; individual or group intervention; and within class or withdrawal styles of administering therapy. Factors relating to the child, such as type and severity of impairment, age, amount of previous therapy and levels of motivation and attention can also influence the outcome of a particular programme of therapy. In addition, intervention usually takes place over an extended period of time and there may be changes to both the child and the service during that time which could positively or negatively affect the outcome. On top of these varied considerations come the decisions regarding the theoretical approach which underpins the method of therapy given and the targets selected.

MRC framework for complex interventions

In evaluating complex interventions such as those used in SLT it is important to use a model which allows for their complex nature. The Medical Research Council (MRC) framework for developing and evaluating complex interventions was first published in 2000 (Campbell, Fitzpatrick, Haines, Kinmouth, Sandercock et al., 2000). This was updated in 2008 (Craig, Dieppe, Macintyre, Michie et al., 2008) and consists of four phases of investigation. The model clarifies that the evaluation process does not progress neatly in a linear fashion, rather the process is iterative; a certain amount of refining and revising at each phase is required before moving to either an earlier or later one.

One difficulty that arises in the evaluation of a complex intervention is that it has not been fully defined or developed. This is accounted for in Phase I, the development phase, where the existing evidence base and current theory are used to underpin the development of the new intervention. During this phase, consideration is given to what type of change is anticipated in response to the intervention and which outcomes might be suited to measure such a change.

Phase II is the feasibility phase, where sampling and recruitment processes are piloted. In this phase, decisions are made regarding what constitutes a change in the behaviour to be modified by the new intervention. This information is needed to help calculate sample size, i.e. what size of sample is needed to detect if a statistically significant change has occurred as a result of the intervention. During this phase, project procedures are tested out and qualitative methods might be used to assess how acceptable the intervention is to those receiving and delivering it.

These first two preparatory phases prepare the ground for a trial at Phase III, the evaluation phase. Here the effectiveness and cost effectiveness of an intervention are examined, generally by conducting a randomized controlled trial.

Finally, Phase IV is the implementation phase. This is where, if appropriate, the intervention is implemented and includes long-term surveillance in order to detect long-term or adverse outcomes that could not be detected in the evaluation phase.

Both the 2000 and 2008 versions of the MRC framework for complex interventions have much of interest to us as clinician–researchers in SLT, and we recommend reading both; they contain summaries, key points and useful questions that the researcher should ask at each stage. Value is given to research at all levels as each individual piece of research builds on previous activity and drives the next stage as we seek to gather more evidence in our profession.

Five phase model of clinical outcome research

Another similar model to the MRC staged framework has been proposed by researchers working specifically within SLT. We recommend you consult this as you embark on your early research activity. Robey and Schultz (1998) proposed a five phase model of clinical outcome research for aphasiologists which was subsequently summarized by Robey in a further publication (see Robey, 2004). Pring (2004) demonstrated how this model could be applied to other areas of intervention research in SLT. The phases are summarized in Table 1.1.

As you start to consider your own research plans, you can identify which level of the model equates to your planned activity. While you might feel that your current activity is at an early stage of the model, it can be helpful to work out what would need to happen after you finish your study to test the findings at a more robust level. Alternatively, if you are thinking about a group trial, it can be helpful to locate the levels for previous work in the field.

Table 1.1 Summary of the five phase model for clinical outcome research advocated by Robey and Schultz (1998).

Phase	Purpose	Achieved by
I	To identify an intervention that has the potential of causing a positive effect and which is not harmful.	Intervention is identified or developed using sound theoretical principles using the existing evidence.
	To carry out small-scale studies to see if the intervention shows a change in behaviour in a positive direction without harmful effects.	Single case studies, case series designs and small group studies.
II	To build on positive findings from phase I and prepare for a phase III trial by: identifying the active component(s) of the intervention, estimating the magnitude of effect that can be considered a clinical change and the optimum dosage to bring this about, identifying the people who will benefit from the intervention and developing inclusion and exclusion criteria to this effect, selecting valid and reliable outcome measures.	As this phase increasingly refines crucial aspects of the study, there may be a progression from hypothesis-testing single case studies to experimental group designs. Increasing specification includes ensuring the intervention is consistent in terms of content and dosage, achieved through manualizing it. Establishing operational definitions for a clinical trial.
III	To obtain stronger evidence that the intervention works by conducting an *efficacy* study. This tests the therapeutic effect of the intervention under *optimal* conditions with the *ideal* sample.	Large-scale randomized controlled trial, gold standard being a parallel groups design.
IV	To assess to what degree the therapeutic effect is realized in day-to-day clinical practice by conducting an *effectiveness* study. This tests the therapeutic effect in *typical* conditions with a *typical* sample.	Expanding the applicability of the original protocol by testing the effects of the intervention when it is delivered in different service delivery models, with specific sub-groups of the target population or testing variants of the original intervention. Hypothesis-testing single case studies to parallel group designs. Conducting meta-analyses of previous studies.
V	Determine who benefits from the intervention and at what cost	Cost-effectiveness studies. Cost-benefit analyses, to assess the benefits in societal terms.

Levels of evidence

The frameworks are also useful tools when considering levels of evidence. As the models portray various stages in the process of evaluating interventions, each is associated with a level of evidence reflecting the relative strength and generalizability of the findings to the population in general. The early stages are associated with weak or low levels of evidence while the 'gold standard', randomized control trial and meta-analysis of systematic reviews, represents the highest or strongest level of evidence. However, this does not mean that the weaker levels of evidence are of less value. Rather, as Pring (2004) points out, these early phases are vital in terms of identifying the specific questions that should be explored within larger scale-research studies. As clinician–researchers, we are ideally placed to carry out early-stage and smaller-scale studies.

The value of small-scale research

As stated above, the focus of this book is to help clinicians gather evidence while carrying out their clinical practice and therefore the focus is mainly on small-scale research. Given the time and resource constraints of clinical practice it is likely that this is more feasible. However, how valuable is small-scale research?

Although the randomized controlled trial (RCT) is considered to be the gold standard of evidence, it also has some drawbacks. By its very nature, it looks for average effects across large populations and does not provide sufficient detail to account for individual differences (see Thompson, 2006). RCTs generally require large numbers of participants to examine the effects of intervention in a powerful way; this might not be possible if the condition is quite rare. Similarly, when researching a population that is varied or heterogeneous, for example people who have acquired aphasia, it may be difficult to recruit sufficient participants to make reliable outcome comparisons across groups.

When evaluating new interventions, as you will see from the models in the previous sections, it is best to start with smaller samples. Small-scale studies therefore have a meaningful role in clinical research; they are usually placed at the beginning of an evaluation of a complex intervention and are a good starting point for those wishing to build evidence-gathering skills. We are aware, however, that having lots of SLTs doing small-scale projects is not necessarily a good way forward in building the evidence base. While the immediate findings might be of interest to us in our clinical setting, they can also be used to drive a larger study at the next phase of the framework. Perhaps, after gaining more research experience you may wish to take your new skills to a higher level of investigation and collaborate with other colleagues to gather evidence on a larger sample, working towards answering the same question. That is not to say we would discourage readers from carrying out larger-scale studies if that is possible and provided they are well supported by a team experienced in research.

Partnering with academic institutions and SLTs working in a research capacity can help us to structure these early phases of research, while considering the possibility of subsequent larger-scale studies. This can be a useful first step for those who want to find an opening into a more research-active career.

How health research is supported in the NHS

Each of the four UK Health Administrations has established clinical research networks and together they form the UK Clinical Research Network (UKCRN). The networks are funded directly by the UK Health Departments. The purpose of the networks and the collaboration between them is to facilitate and support high-quality research for the benefit of patients by providing an infrastructure. The networks work together to develop and coordinate UK-wide initiatives and provide opportunities for patients and staff to engage in research projects. Strategic health authorities are required to demonstrate that NHS trusts work with the clinical research networks in order to contribute to the increase of health service research, which can then feed back into clinical practice for the benefit of those using the NHS. Support and training are available through these networks, which deliver high-quality research in the UK. Each of the UK countries has different arrangements for supporting clinical research under the umbrella of the UKCRN. See the website in the Research Support section at the end of this chapter to find out more about the networks in your particular country.

The NIHR clinical research network portfolio and how it could help you

The NIHR portfolio is a public database of clinical research studies which are defined by their presence on that list as being high quality. Studies funded by the NIHR and its partner organizations, such as the MRC and some charitable organizations such as the Stroke Association and Cancer Research UK are automatically eligible for the portfolio, and others can be adopted too if they meet the defined quality criteria. Studies which appear on the portfolio are eligible to be considered for support by the Clinical Research Network.

You can search the portfolio to see if your potential research project is already being undertaken by someone else. In addition, it could be the gateway to gaining some experience in research; new and on-going projects often wish to recruit participants from other sites to ensure their sample population is large enough, so you can be part of a larger project by recruiting people locally for it.

You can find the NIHR portfolio on the NIHR website and enter details of clinical areas you are interested in such as stroke, communication problems, services, etc. This will lead you to the various studies that are currently being conducted in the UK in those fields. You will see from the details of each study if they are recruiting participants. If they are, then you can request further information and a study protocol from the researching team. After reading the protocol, if you are interested in taking part and have the sort of clinical caseload that could support recruitment into the study, you can then formally apply to join it as a recruiting site. Organizations (NHS trusts) whose researchers recruit patients into NIHR portfolio studies receive funding from their Local Comprehensive Network, and this is invested into infrastructure to deliver research. There are local variations of how this is managed, and your R&D office can provide you with more information. This is an ideal way to get started in research; the planning and protocol have already been written and this will give you an insight into how research operates before you embark on your own study; of course, you will need to discuss this with your manager and your R&D department before committing to recruiting participants. It will also bring funds for research into your trust so your R&D department could be pleased to support you.

If you decide to get involved in an existing study through the NIHR portfolio, then, depending on the type of study, you could be delivering a novel therapy or gathering information about your clients. Whatever you are required to do you will strictly follow the study protocol that has been developed by those who are heading the research. Your R&D department will be able to give you more information about recruiting for such studies and help you with any questions you may have. Some R&D departments actively search for studies for their employees to engage in, as this allows the organization to continue to invest in research infrastructure to deliver research and improve outcomes in their services, whilst raising the profile of the organization as a research active trust.

Good Clinical Practice (GCP)

Good Clinical Practice (GCP) refers to the code of conduct for NHS research which should be followed and which is monitored through research governance. Although the name suggests 'clinical' practice, it is in fact referring to good practice in clinical research. All clinical research in the UK must comply with these guidelines and it is expected that at least one member of each research team will have received training in GCP. In practice, it is better if all members have attended such training.

The guidelines seek to protect participants and promote high-quality research through ensuring that, among other things, adequate risk assessments have been carried out, information and consent arrangements for participants are adhered to, sound protocols are developed and followed throughout the research, and data is protected and adequately stored.

The Local Research Networks and some R&D departments provide training on GCP, so researchers can be aware of the protocols they need to adhere to. Ask your R&D department about this. As a minimum you may be required to undertake a day's training or follow an online course in how to take consent, for example. See the Resources section for more information on this.

Public and Patient Involvement (PPI)

The involvement of the public in making decisions about health care management is also a crucial element in clinical research, and one of the elements on which an application for funding will be judged is the level and appropriateness of PPI in your proposal. Our patients can be involved at every stage of the research process. For example, they are a rich source of ideas and outcome measures for investigation, can offer you opinions on the presentation of information sheets (particularly important when involving people who have communication difficulties), can give you a patient's perspective on logistical issues that might affect your project, and can be involved in the dissemination of your findings. You will find PPI referred to throughout the book.

Approval processes

As research engages participants in something that is generating new knowledge and is not part of normal service delivery, a number of approvals are required before it can be carried out, particularly in the NHS. These include a positive ethical opinion and Research and Development (R&D) approval (also known as NHS permission). Ethical review is carried out in order to assess the level of risk to participants and researchers when engaging in the project and to ensure that the interests of the participants are considered throughout the research process; R&D approval ensures the project will be adequately supported by funding, expertise and realistic timescales. Each research project carried out in the NHS will also require a sponsor, whose job it is to ensure it can be managed adequately in terms of safety, finances, data integrity, etc. and that it can be supported at the site selected. Sponsorship should be in place before a project proceeds for ethical review and R&D approval. Chapters 2 and 3 give further information about approval processes, and each of the chapters in Part II of the book deals with particular ethical issues you might face in trying to answer a question similar to that in the chapter title. The R&D department in your trust or institution will also be able to help you.

Service evaluation and audit do not require R&D or NHS ethical approvals since they do not generate new knowledge about a particular approach or views of people or relationships that occur, but provide information about the standards that the existing service achieves. However, depending on where you are conducting the research, you may need University ethical approval and it is still good clinical practice to gain consent if you wish to conduct a service evaluation and, for example, want to gain the views and experiences of your patients.

Research in the context of the WHO ICF

The World Health Organisation's (WHO) International Classification of Function, Disability and Health (ICF) (World Health Organisation, 2007) is a framework for addressing healthcare. It was recognized that, in the past, healthcare has mainly been directed at managing health problems at the level of bodily structure and function and has failed to address the broader impact of illness upon the person. The framework does this by including the impact of the impairment/illness on activity and participation, environmental aspects that can influence a person's adaptation or recovery and also personal and societal factors. For more information on the application of the WHO ICF to communication disorders, see Threats (2008) and Ma, Threats and Worrall (2008).

SLTs are being encouraged to use this framework when carrying out clinical management, and a number of studies have reported the use of the ICF in terms of taking a holistic approach to our understanding of communication impairment and its effect on quality of life (McCormack, McAllister, McLeod, & Harrison, 2012; Miller, Noble, Jones, & Burn, 2006; Yorkston, Klasner, & Swanson, 2001). There is also an increasing awareness of the need to consider children's views as evidenced by the publication of the edited book by Roulstone and McLeod (2011).

Naturally, research in these broader areas require suitable outcome measures and a number of researchers have been developing these (see Walshe, Peach & Miller, 2009; Hilari, Lamping, Smith, Northcott, Lamb, & Marshall, 2009; Long, Hesketh, Paszek, Booth, & Bowen, 2008). Such assessments are a boon to the new researcher wishing to investigate how communication impairment and our interventions impact upon these aspects of activity and participation.

Summary

This chapter lays out the context for practice-based evidence. It defines and differentiates types of evidence and explains what drives, guides, promotes and supports research in the NHS. It also shows how small-scale research fits within the models for evaluating complex interventions.

This background information will prepare you for reading the rest of Part I and relevant chapters in Parts II and III. These chapters will help you to gather evidence by guiding you in setting up the process involved. They will also make you aware of what support you might need, where to find it and what information to have ready when you seek advice. They will get you to think critically, not only about others' work but also your own, so you can feel confident that you have done a thorough job. They will also provide useful resources and suggestions for further, more detailed reading.

You may be reading this book for your personal and professional development or because you have been asked to provide evidence about what you do for someone else; the following chapters will guide you in gathering practice-based evidence, whether it be working towards a future career in research or feeling more confident in demonstrating and justifying what you do.

References

Campbell, M., Fitzpatrick, R., Haines, A., Kinmonth, A., Sandercock, P., Spiegelhalter, D., & Tyrer, P. (2000) Framework for design and evaluation of complex interventions to improve health. *British Medical Journal* **321**, 694–696.

Craig, P., Dieppe, P., Macintyre, S., Michie, S., Nazareth, I., & Petticrew, M. (2008) *Developing and Evaluating Complex Interventions: New Guidance*. Medical Research Council. www.mrc.ac.uk/complexinterventionsguidance

Dollaghan, C. A. (2007) *The Handbook for Evidence Based Practice in Communication Disorders*. Baltimore: Paul H Brookes.

Hilari, K., Lamping, D. L., Smith, S. C., Northcott, S., Lamb, A., & Marshall, J. (2009) Psychometric properties of the Stroke and Aphasia Quality of Life Scale (SAQOL-39) in a generic stroke population. *Clinical Rehabilitation* **23:6**, 544–557.

Long. A. F., Hesketh, A., Paszek, G., Booth, M., & Bowen, A. (2008) Development of a reliable self-report outcome measure for pragmatic trials of communication therapy following stroke: The Communication Outcome after Stroke (COAST) scale. *Clinical Rehabilitation* **22:12**, 1083–1094.

Ma, E. P-M., Threats, T. T., & Worrall, L. E. (2008) An introduction to the International Classification of Functioning, Disability and Health (ICF) for speech-language pathology: Its past, present and future. *International Journal of Speech-Language Pathology* **10**, 2–8.

McCormack, J., McAllister, L., McLeod, S. & Harrison, L. (2012) Knowing, having, doing: The battles of childhood speech impairment. *Child Language Teaching and Therapy* **28:2**, 141–157.

Miller, N., Noble, E., Jones, D., & Burn, D. (2006) Life with communication changes in Parkinson's Disease. *Age and Ageing* **35:3**, 235–239.

Pring, T. (2004) Ask a silly question: Two decades of troublesome trials. *International Journal of Language and Communication Disorders* **39:3**, 285–302.

Robey, R. R. (2004) A five-phase model for clinical outcome research. *Journal of Communication Disorders* **37**, 401–411.

Robey, R. R. and Schulz, M. C. (1998) A model for conducting clinical-outcome research: An adaptation of the standard protocol for use in Aphasiology. *Aphasiology* **12**, 787–810.

Roulstone, S. E. and McLeod, S. (Eds) (2011) *Listening to Children and Young People with Speech, Language and Communication Needs*. Guildford: J&R Press.

Royal College of Speech and Language Therapists (2009) *The RCSLT Research Strategy*. http://www.rcslt.org/members/research/intro

Thompson, C. K. (2006) Single subject controlled experiments in aphasia: The science and state of the science. *Journal of Communication Disorders* **39:4**, 266–291.

Threats, T. T. (2006) Towards an international framework for communication disorders: Use of the ICF. *Journal of Communication Disorders* **39:4**, 251–265.

Walshe, M., Peach, R. K., & Miller, N. (2009) Dysarthria Impact Profile: Development of a scale to measure psychosocial effects. *International Journal of Language and Communication Disorders* **44:5**, 693–715.

World Health Organisation (2007) *International Classification of Functioning, Disability and Health.* http://www.who.int/classifications/icf/

Yorkston, K., Klasner, E., and Swanson, K. (2001) Communication in context: A qualitative study of the experiences of individuals with multiple sclerosis. *American Journal of Speech-Language Pathology* **10:2**, 126–137.

Further reading

Moule, P. and Hek, G. (2011) *Making Sense of Research: An Introduction for Health and Social Care Practitioners* (4th edition). London: Sage Publications.

Roddam, H. and Skeat, G. (Eds) (2010) *Embedding Evidence-Based Practice in Speech and Language Therapy: International Examples.* Chichester: Wiley-Blackwell.

Special editions on the ICF and communication disorders:

International Journal of Speech-Language Pathology (2008) **10:1–2**. Special edition: Contributions of the ICF to speech-language pathology.

Seminars in Speech and Language (2007) **28:4**, Special edition on the ICF.

Resources

Hutchinson, D. (2009) *12 Golden GCP Rules for Investigators* (3rd edition). Guildford: Canary Ltd.

The Institute of Clinical Research (1996) *ICH Harmonised Tripartite Guideline for Good Clinical Practice.* IFPMA, Switzerland.

National Patient Safety Agency, National Research Ethics Service (2007) *Defining Research*, **Issue 3**

Research support

Royal College of Speech and Language Therapists: provides details of the RCSLT research strategy and other useful information relating to research in SLT. http://www.rcslt.org

National Institute of Health Research: this website provides details of studies in the NIHR portfolio, access to the UK Research Networks and details of funding opportunities amongst other useful information. http://www.nihr.ac.uk

UK Clinical Research Networks (UKCRN): this website provides information about the UK clinical research networks. http://www.ukcrc.org/infrastructure/networks/

2 The process of gathering evidence

Sue Roulstone and Rosemarie Hayhow

Learning outcomes

By the end of this chapter, you will be able to:

- Reflect on your current practice in order to identify areas in which you need evidence to support or develop your practice
- Identify the existing knowledge around your chosen area
- Develop a question that is feasible and will produce useful findings
- Turn your question into a detailed plan
- Manage your data collection, organization and storage
- Make sense of your data
- Develop a protocol to guide your investigation

Introduction

This chapter provides a template for constructing a plan to develop practice-based evidence. It presents a series of stages to consider in the development of evidence. These are set out specifically with practice-based evidence in mind and can be used with a range of research activity from small-scale investigative studies to more formal trials. In Part II of the book, authors follow this general template to address clinical research questions that generate different types of evidence.

Although presented in this chapter as a linear process, it is often necessary to proceed in a more iterative fashion. In practice, information acquired as you go along feeds back into your thinking and planning. It is rare when planning a study to be able to progress relentlessly from one stage to the next. Frequently, we need time and other information to progress our thinking. This can mean that we need to go back and repeat stages in the light of our new insights and information and the process is therefore iterative rather than linear. Figure 2.1 sets out the suggested process and the following sections expand on each of the numbered steps. We set out the purpose of each stage, explaining what each aims to achieve, and then provide some suggestions for action which will lead to the development of your research protocol (see section below).

Generally, when developing practice-based evidence, it is likely that your investigation will be at the level of developing the theory of an intervention or showing that the intervention has a potentially active component rather than running a large-scale trial of its effectiveness (Medical Research Council, 2008). Start with something that feels manageable and in which you can develop your skills and build up experience with support.

It is necessary to involve service users at all stages of the process so that our investigations are relevant to both professionals and users. The people who use speech and language therapy services see them from a very different perspective to the professional who delivers the service and could have different priorities. Additionally, some of our users have been using services for a long time through many stages of their lives and have a longer perspective than the professionals. The involvement of service users in research is usually known as Public and Patient Involvement or PPI.

1. What are the clinical issues or challenges?

Purpose: to reflect on your current practice in order to identify areas in which you need to find or create evidence to support or develop your practice.

The motivation to embark on developing practice-based evidence may have come from a number of directions: from managers or commissioners who need us to justify our services; from the people and families who need to understand the reasons behind decisions; from our own motivation to improve a particular aspect of our work; from the need to work out what action to take in a difficult or unusual case. In our daily practice, there could be many areas that need practice-based evidence. Here are some techniques to help identify and prioritize one that you can take forward.

Actions

- Write down all the clinical decisions you have made today. For each one, identify the evidence that underpins that decision. You might be able to identify a particular study, a theory or an author or there may be a gap in the evidence.

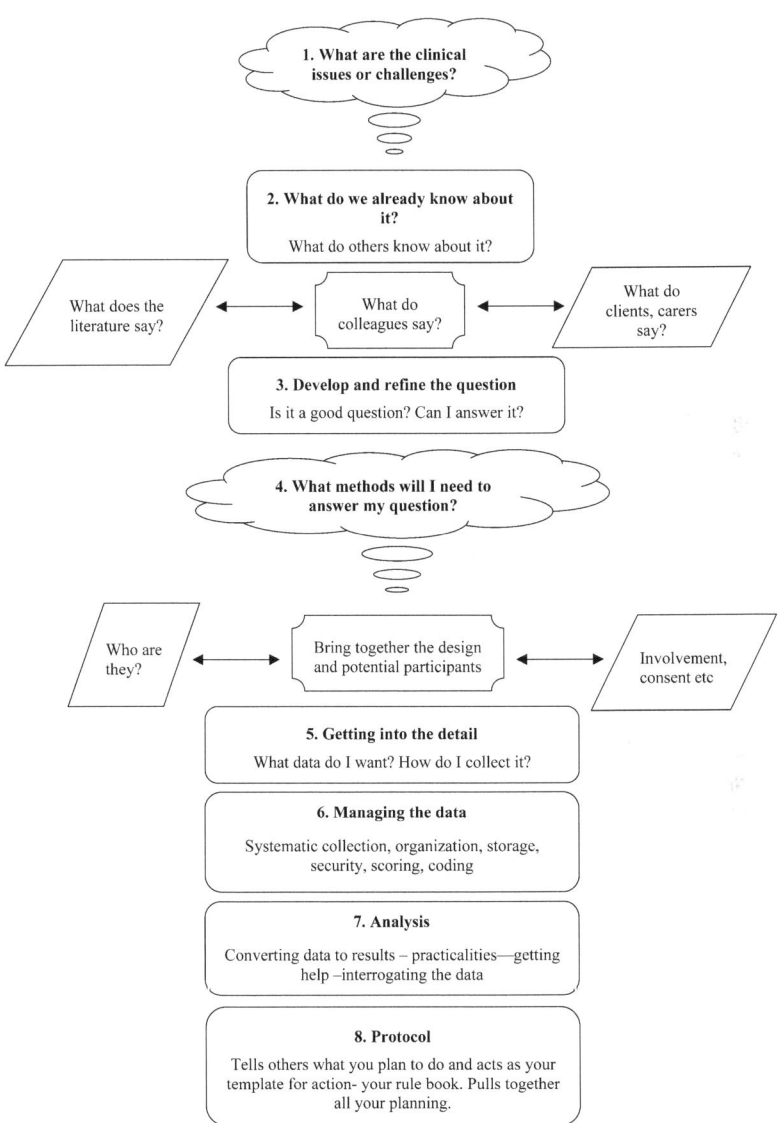

Figure 2.1 The process of gathering evidence.

- Make a list of new ideas that you have had recently, or new developments that you made to your practice. Then identify what you know about the existing evidence that supports your ideas or changes to practice and identify gaps in the evidence that underpins them.

- Think about your most difficult case in the last week and identify what information or evidence might have helped you to deal more effectively with that case. Check with your users: the issues that challenge you may not be relevant to your users; they may have other burning questions about the service or interventions. They may have a view regarding the most important questions or the sorts of issues that will have the most impact on their quality of life.

When we are seeking support from management to conduct investigations or evaluations of a topic or problem, it could help if it is perceived to be valuable by our service users. Most health providers now have patient advisory groups who support patient involvement and communication (Patient and Public Involvement officers). Your department might wish to set up its own service advisory group, by routinely telling all new patients about the group and inviting participation. There might also be a related disease-specific group such as a stroke group, or one of your existing parent groups that might agree to discuss ideas for research with you. It is important that these conversations are conducted ethically; that is, that the service user understands the nature and purpose of the discussion and has consented, without coercion, to participate.

Although one issue might already stand out as the most urgent or important, the likelihood is that this process generates lots of gaps where you need practice-based evidence. Prioritize one by determining which would be most useful to you, to your clients, to your manager or to the commissioners of your service.

2. What do we already know about it?

Purpose: to identify the existing knowledge around your chosen issue.
As you embark on developing practice-based evidence, it is vital to find out what knowledge already exists about the issue you want to investigate. It is possible that some practitioners/researchers have already developed good evidence in this area so future work may need to refocus or build on their work. Others could have tackled something similar and you might be able to learn from their methods – and their mistakes. Someone else may have identified the issue as

important and there could be an opportunity to collaborate. There might also be individuals with expertise in the methods needed to explore this area or in the theoretical ideas that can help you to design your study.

Service users are often experts in their own condition and aware of the latest research, so it is important to tap into the knowledge base of patient groups.

Actions

- *The literature*: there are a number of review sites available which may help you to find existing studies and relevant research (see Further Reading). These sites provide searchable databases which focus on literature which has been quality assured. This means that the studies have been evaluated for the robustness and appropriateness of the methods used. If there is no review available that is relevant to your topic, then the librarians within the local trust, university or city libraries can help to carry out a literature search. Chapter 3 provides more detail on the process of literature searching and tips to help you with this stage.

- *Colleagues and subject experts*: although we may feel tentative about exploring ideas with recognized experts, an important part of developing an idea is to expose it to the views of others. Before approaching colleagues, work out some specific questions, have a clear agenda and consider what might motivate a colleague to support you. For example, you could offer to share the output of your literature search with them, or you might be able to recruit some of their patients for your study.

- *Service users and third sector:* third sector organizations such as Afasic, the Stroke Association, the British Stammering Association and the Communication Trust have often published summaries of evidence. Check their websites and also those of local service user organizations.

- *Write up your review:* gather all your reading together in a written summary. The process of writing can help you to think through and develop your ideas. This summary may also come in useful if you need to write a report, or if you need to explain your study to others. It will also form the background to your protocol (see Section 8).

3. Refining the question

Purpose: to develop a question that is feasible and will produce useful findings.

When developing practice-based evidence, your initial idea will probably be quite broad. However, to generate a project that is feasible, useful, interesting and ethical, it is necessary to progressively refine the question. A well-defined question will drive the rest of your investigation. This stage is usually iterative and interacts with the previous one in that your discussions, reading and writing will be part of what helps to refine the question or questions. The process involved is one of increasing specification. Two examples are given below that show how a general aim can be increasingly specified.

Actions

(a) Write down your overall aim.

(b) Now try to break that down into more and more specific objectives. Specific objectives will further define your area of interest and help towards refining your question.

Example 1. If your overall aim is to evaluate parental or carer involvement, this might translate into various objectives, for example: to describe key components of parent or carer involvement from their perspective; to investigate parent/spouse preferences for sessions with or without their children/spouse present; to assess changes in parents' knowledge and skills following parents' involvement sessions; to compare the number of treatment sessions required to achieve objectives with and without parent/carer involvement.

Example 2. If your overall aim is to evaluate the impact of your therapy, this might translate into the objectives: to evaluate the effect of phonological awareness therapy on children's speech; to evaluate the impact of conversation groups on patient's self esteem and confidence; to evaluate the effect of vocabulary therapy on patients/children's language.

(c) Now take your objective and turn it into a question.

Example 1. The objective 'to describe key components of parental or carer involvement from their perspective' might lead to the question: What do parents or carers perceive to be the most important aspects of their involvement in therapy?

Example 2. The objective 'to evaluate the effects of vocabulary therapy on patients'/children's language' might be rephrased as the question: Does vocabulary therapy improve the word finding performance of patients/children?

(d) Now take each component, or concept within that question, and define it.

Example 1. The question is: What do <u>parents or carers</u> <u>perceive</u> to be the most important aspects of their <u>involvement in therapy</u>?

By defining the underlined components of the question, a more specific version emerges that will help us to plan the next stage of investigation.

<u>Parents</u>: does this mean mothers and fathers? What about grandparents or other carers who might bring the child to sessions?

<u>Carers</u>: do you mean the person who spends the most time with the patient or do you really mean the patient's spouse/partner?

Are there particular sectors of the population you wish to include – for example, parents/carers living in particular areas or parents/carers from a particular background? Will the study focus on all the parents/carers in the service or those associated with particular groups of children or adults – of a certain age group or diagnostic category?

<u>Perceive</u>: this suggests an interest in what the parents/carers think about their involvement rather than what the professional might think is their view and therefore points to a particular approach to asking the questions (see methods, next section).

<u>Involvement in therapy</u>: which therapy will the study focus on? Is there a problem with a particular type of intervention or is this a more general question about all types of involvement across the service?

Example 2. The question is: Does <u>vocabulary therapy</u> <u>improve</u> the <u>word finding performance</u> of <u>patients/children</u>?

By defining the underlined components of the question in this way, we can identify a more specific version that will help us to plan the next stage of investigation.

Vocabulary therapy: does this include all approaches to vocabulary therapy or is a very particular approach being evaluated; who is delivering the therapy and how frequently?

Improve: what will you recognize as improvement? How much change counts as valuable change? From whose perspective are you judging the improvement – the therapists' perspective or that of the client or their family or from the perspective of people like teachers and other significant people in the patient's circle?

Word finding performance: how will we measure word finding and in what social and linguistic contexts?

Patients/children: does the question need to focus on a particular age group or diagnostic group of patients/children, or in those with a particular social or linguistic background? Is there interest in patients/children in a particular clinic site or across all sites and client groups in your service?

For a question that focuses on the evaluation of an intervention, the evidence-based practice literature suggests a similar process whereby the mnemonic PICO (see http://www.cebm.net/) is used to focus questions about intervention (Participants, the Intervention, the Comparison intervention and the Outcome of interest). So, in determining the effectiveness of an intervention, it is first necessary to define who will be the **participants** in the study and which **intervention** will be evaluated. You also need to define the **comparison** intervention – will there be a non-intervention control or are you comparing to a standard care package or to another specified intervention.

Finally, it is necessary to specify the main **outcome** that will be measured to show an effect. Chapter 8 provides an example of this.

A statement of your overall aim and your specific research question now needs to be written into your protocol (see Section 8).

4. What methods will I need to answer my question?

Purpose: to reflect on the nature of the question that is being asked in order to consider the implications for the methods you might use.

It is important that the research strategy that is employed is appropriate to the question being asked. In broad terms, we can make a distinction between quantitative and qualitative strategies. Bryman (2008) explains the practical differences between the two strategies: if we are interested in the views of a particular group of people, we are more likely to choose a qualitative strategy that allows us to explore how participants interpret their world. If, on the other hand, we are interested in working out which is the most important source of variation between different individuals or groups, then a quantitative strategy is more likely to fit the question. If we already have a well-developed hypothesis to test, then a quantitative strategy is likely to be appropriate. If, however, there is little theory or pre-existing research about our question, then a qualitative approach may be more useful.

In some cases, you might wish to measure a particular variable and at the same time explore people's perspectives on a complementary aspect, in which case a mixed methods strategy that combines quantitative and qualitative methods may then be appropriate. Finally, if your question is more in the form of a problem to be solved, an action research strategy may be useful. For example, if you are unhappy with an aspect of your practice and want to change it, you might collaborate with others to decide on how the practice should be changed and how you monitor that change. Your methods of data collection when using an action research strategy may be either quantitative and/or qualitative.

A little reminder about the term 'qualitative': sometimes we read of analyses that describe the nature of a particular problem. For example, people will talk about quantitative and qualitative analyses of stammering; this usually means that they are counting stammers for a quantitative analysis and describing the type of stammer (a block or a repetition) for the qualitative analysis. However, this use of 'qualitative' is in contrast to how the term is used in the research literature, where the term refers to research which investigates a phenomenon or experience from the perspective of the participant.

There are a number of scenarios below, each asking a different kind of question. The nature of the question determines the kind of data that you are looking for – whether you are trying to measure something (quantitative) or explore experiences or views (qualitative). Read each one in order to help you understand the differences between qualitative and quantitative data. Then work out which type of strategy best fits your own question.

Actions

- Do you want to explore people's explanations about their feelings on a topic or do you want to measure their feelings on some kind of scale? If you are doing the former and have no set or pre-existing ideas (or no *a priori* theory) about how these people feel and want to learn about their perspective, this is best answered using a qualitative approach. This may in turn lead you to interview people individually or in groups (see Chapter 6 for more information on investigating people's perspectives). Alternatively, if you want to quantify people's feelings, it suggests that you already have some ideas about their perspective and have a scale that fits your ideas, or an existing theory about how they might feel. This is a quantitative approach and will lead to a questionnaire or survey.

▪ Perhaps you have been asked to produce evidence about the range of children that pass through your service or you may need to find out if parents have any problems with your service and what these are. The first issue is likely to generate descriptive data, numbers of children in different age groups or diagnostic categories and will therefore follow a quantitative strategy (see Chapter 8 for more information on collecting data on numbers). For the second issue, you have no way of predicting their view, so will need to generate opinions and views collected through interviews or focus groups. In this case, a qualitative strategy is more appropriate.

▪ It might be that you need to produce some outcome data for a particular clinic or client group. Some of this might be quantitative data in that you need to be able to show change scores on certain parameters of language and communication, such as the percentage of syllables stuttered or the percentage of consonants correct (see Chapter 4 for more information on measuring the effects of intervention on impairment). This would be a quantitative strategy. However, you may also feel that information about how patients or families perceive any changes will provide an important perspective on the outcomes; this may require a qualitative strategy. Providing data using both strategies comprises a mixed method strategy (Glogowska, 2011) and you will need to give particular thought as to how you present both types of data in a robust fashion.

5. Getting into the detail

Purpose: this stage is about developing a detailed plan of action from your question. This plan will be consistent with your selected methodology and take account of the specifics of your question, your context and the people you have identified as potential participants. Detailed planning is required for a study to run smoothly and to meet the necessary approvals, which means you need to think carefully about all the details. Time spent in the planning stage will save you time and frustration in the longer term.

Preliminaries

Purpose: to find information to help with planning the detail. Throughout, we are describing the stages in designing your project as if it is a linear process, but this is far from the case. For example, you need to do quite a bit of thinking about what you want to do before you can seek help from research design services or support from Research and Development (R&D) personnel. However, don't leave it too long before you speak to someone and get advice.

You need to work out whether or not you require ethics approval for your study. In this chapter, we are limiting ourselves to the processes required in the UK but the requirements are similar wherever you are working. Although the details of the processes and the available support will vary, the underlying principles are widely accepted and apply to research in a variety of settings.

Actions

Training in research governance: there is increasing requirement on anyone who is responsible for running a study, who takes participant consent and is involved in other research activities with participants to have formal training in these processes. In the UK, such courses are known as Good Clinical Practice or GCP courses. This is a rather misleading phrase as it refers to the practice of clinical research rather than the clinical skills and practice that are part and parcel of our everyday working lives. R&D departments have information on approved courses.

Ethics and R&D approval: two key sources are available to you to help identify what approvals you will need for your study.

- Visit the National Research Ethics Service (NRES) website (http://www.nres.npsa.nhs.uk/home):

  Download the documents (NRES, 2011) that will help you work out whether your study is research, evaluation, or audit; then look at some of the templates so that you can see what is required in participant information sheets, consent forms, etc. These are useful to look at even if your study is not going to require ethics approval. You can also read their guidance on confidentiality and other issues that are relevant to your study.

- Visit the Research and Development (R&D) department's pages on your employer's website.

Look at the researcher guidelines and the documents they need in order to evaluate the following: participant safety, confidentiality, the participant consenting process, funding and costs to your employer, and the practicalities of your study. Do they indicate funding opportunities that could apply to your study? Note the name and contact details of the staff member who you should contact to discuss your study. Once you have decided on what you plan to do, arrange a meeting to talk it through with them. You can also visit the NHS R&D forum website (http://www.rdforum.nhs.uk) to see if there is any further information that is helpful to you at this stage.

Once you have worked on the details of your project, you are closer to working on your ethics or R&D application and to think if there are any risks or costs for your participants. Chapter 3 gives further details on approvals processes. Even if you do not need formal NHS ethics approval for your study, there are useful resources on the NRES website which will help you ensure that your participants are giving informed consent.

It is essential that we are honest about why we are doing a study and that participants understand what it involves, which means we must be able to describe it in different ways for different participants. You need to write, in lay terms, your purpose and what your study involves; this is good practice even when ethics approval is not required. Firstly, write it for a parent/carer or adult client with no comprehension impairment. Then, if children are to be involved, write it for a child of the appropriate age and think about how you will ask them to consent and how they will indicate this. Consider a different format for children or adults with comprehension and expressive difficulties, for example, pictures with minimal text or pictures with a spoken explanation. Consult users, parents and carers and refer to the literature for strategies and techniques that have been tried and tested with children or vulnerable adults. You may have colleagues with relevant experience who can help you develop the resources you need (see Merrick, 2011 for a discussion of assent/consent with children and young people with speech, language and communication difficulties).

If your study will involve schools or other non-NHS settings you will need to satisfy their requirements. Usually, the robustness of the NHS procedures satisfies other academic or educational governance and ethics procedures and so it is matter of cooperation rather than duplication.

Detailed planning

Purpose: now we build on the work you have done so far on refining your question, defining the components of your question and choosing your methodology. Return to your refined research question (Section 3) with the definitions of the concepts or components that you developed. Were you specific enough to now elaborate the details? We will consider some of the finer details in relation to participants, intervention or experiences of an intervention and outcome.

Participants: at this point, you need to consider precisely who your participants should be, how you will access or generate a pool of potential participants and how you will select them.

- Can you work with a small group of users to hear their ideas about how best to engage your participants?

- What sampling procedures will you use? You could advertise your study and invite participants to contact you so that you have a **self-selected** sample. Alternatively, invite everyone who is referred to your clinic or on your caseload who meet your criteria – this would be a **convenience** sample. Another option would be to define a very specific range of participants in terms of: age; severity of problem; time since onset/ diagnosis; or gender mix so that your sample has a similar distribution to that of the specific communication impairment. This will give you a **representative** sample. Finally, you could sample across a range of factors that you think will have an impact on the kind of question you are asking for a **purposive** sample.

- What are your inclusion and exclusion criteria? This will further clarify your participants. You might use specific baseline measures to ensure that participants all meet your specified criteria or use broader criteria like age and SLT diagnosis.

- How many participants do you need? This will depend upon the nature of your study and the methodology you are using and, crucially, upon the context in which the study will take place. If you plan a quantitative study then discussion with someone with statistical experience of similar studies may be helpful at this point. If your question concerns the perceptions of your users, it may be qualitative in nature and need only a small number of participants.

Types of investigation

There are a range of types of investigation you might want to carry out.

If you are studying a specific intervention, you will need to consider details such as length and frequency of the treatment sessions, how long a treatment episode will be, what the key components of the intervention are and how the intervention can be delivered in a consistent way. This may be clearly described in a manual or it could be an approach that you and your colleagues have developed and documented. If you don't already have a clear description of your intervention, consider using a framework such as that described by McCauley and Fey (2006) which sets out the components of an intervention. You will also need to decide what your outcomes will be and how you will measure them.

If you are interested in people's views of your service, then you might want to consider using a questionnaire with a combination of closed questions and free-text. Alternatively, you may first conduct some interviews or a focus group to identify key issues which you can then incorporate into your questionnaire.

If you are interested in people's experiences of an intervention or of living with a particular communication impairment, you might use qualitative methods and will need to consider how much structure you will impose on your interviews workshops, focus groups or any other context that you plan using for your data collection (Guion, Diehl, & McDonald, 2011; Turner, 2010; Kvale, 1996). If the communication impairment or age of participants make it difficult to obtain the sort of in-depth data usually required of a qualitative study, could you use other or additional mediums for obtaining some insight into your participants' experiences? (See Roulstone & McLeod, 2011, for ways of obtaining the perspectives of children and young people.)

For more information on these and other types of investigation, see the chapters in Part II.

Throughout this phase of 'getting into the detail' your current patients and others with relevant experience are a valuable resource. The NHS National

Institute for Health Research (NIHR) and the charity INVOLVE, which focuses on public engagement, both have a wealth of information and expertise about public and patient involvement (PPI). Their websites are listed in the Resources section at the end of this chapter.

Logistics

You will need to sort out the practical aspects of your study such as where you might see your participants, how you will set up any assessments you plan to do, whether you have the right equipment and if you need any administration support for setting up focus groups or transcription, etc. For more information on this, see Chapter 3 and each of the relevant chapters in Part II.

The level and quantity of detail your study requires will clearly vary with, among other things, the complexity of what you are doing, the number of participants you hope to engage and the extent of divergence from your normal clinical practice that your study entails. Careful planning of the details will help you write your protocol and make the transition from ideas to practicalities, from concepts to activities and materials.

6. Managing the data

Purpose: to develop systematic data collection and storage procedures so that you collect all that you need, can access the dataset easily and ensure that material or anything that would lead to the identification of participants is kept confidential and secure.

Security and confidentiality are an important part of clinical work and the issues for any study or project are similar. Data, like treatment notes, must be accurately recorded and checks should be in place to identify errors. Whatever the nature of your data, there will be software to help with organization, storing, coding and analysis. You may need to work with your IT department so that you can make full use of the freely-available software that can support research studies while maintaining confidentiality. Ethics Committees and Information Governance Officers assess planned data collection and storage processes, and will want to know for how long you need to keep the data and what you plan to do with it at the end of your study.

Collecting data is usually one of the interesting and enjoyable stages of a project but, when it is done as part of a busy clinical day, it is easy to fall behind in managing that data. There is often quite a lot of work to be done to organize your data (whether it is quantitative or qualitative) before you can begin your analysis, and it is best to do this as soon as possible after you have collected the data. Trying to document your data collection processes or transcribe data days or weeks after it has been collected can be difficult – remembering details of the process in retrospect will be tricky. So having clear plans for managing your data before you start will help you keep on top of these tasks. Systematic data management is good research practice and essential for researcher sanity. See Chapter 3 for more details on data storage.

Actions:

- Ensure that you have a lockable filing cabinet for raw data and that you can create password-protected files for computer storage of identifiable data.

- If it is necessary for you to anonymize, then you need to keep the identifying 'key' separate to the research files. Work out a system for identifying your participants when you separate data from names.

- Quantitative and demographic data can be organized on spreadsheets or put straight into statistical analysis software.

- Free text, where responses are complex and diverse, can be stored as text for a future thematic analysis; where the responses are simple and straightforward, you may be able to carry out some content codings directly into a spreadsheet.

- Transcripts of qualitative data need organizing too. Labelling speakers clearly and consistently and assigning page, line or paragraph numbers ensure that you can refer back easily to the original source of a quote or for examples of a particular code.

Data management and data analysis are closely linked and often it is difficult to determine where one stops and the other starts. This is particularly true for qualitative data where your initial coding helps you organize your data into the themes that inform your analysis. It is helpful to think about the stages of qualitative analysis (for example, Braun & Clark, 2006) before deciding how you will organize your data so that there is consistency between your chosen systems for management and analysis. This will help you consider the best way to keep track of and organize the many codes that will make up your coding system. You could opt for the tried-and-tested index cards, paper and post-it system. You could cut and paste into tables using your usual word processing software. Alternatively, you might be interested in learning how to use software designed to assist qualitative analysis. If this appeals to you, visit the Computer Assisted Qualitative Data AnalysiS (CAQDAS) networking project where there is information about different packages, training courses and much more. These decisions will depend upon the size and number of your samples, your resources and working preferences as well as upon the recommended procedures for your particular sort of analysis.

Finally, plan a way to check the accuracy of your data systems. For example, enter some of your numerical data twice and crosscheck for accuracy; ask a colleague to transcribe a sample independently or read through your transcript whilst listening to the sample.

Once you have worked through these points you will have the detail required for your protocol showing that you will run your study efficiently while safeguarding participant confidentiality. You may also have identified additional support or training that you need.

7. Analysis

Purpose: to make sense of the data you have collected and find out if you have answered your research question.
This is where it gets really exciting. Has your intervention made a difference? Have you gained insights into the experiences of clients or carers? Have you identified a treatment factor that seems important to overall outcome? This is where all your work from the very beginning of the process to this stage comes together.

Organization and analysis run closely together. Well-organized data is much quicker and easier to analyse.

In general, what you do with your data depends upon your research questions, your methods and the type of data you have collected. If you are using quantitative methods and plan to collect numerical data, then you can describe the range, the averages and the differences. You may also want to analyze your data using more formal statistical methods. Depending on your level of familiarity with these, you might wish to seek the advice of a statistician.

If you plan to collect qualitative data, then you will need to 'code' the ideas, concepts, terms, etc. and then begin to look for themes and patterns. These themes may be more abstract or they may organize into hierarchies.

Although you must keep returning to the transcripts you are also working with your codes and analyzing them. This stage can be referred to as *analytic or theoretical coding* as your experience and knowledge begins to interact with your data to arrive at new understandings. You may find that your qualitative data takes you to new areas of literature as your participants' experiences open up different ways of looking at events.

At this stage, you still need to keep an eye on the detail, but you need also to put this detail into a larger perspective, relating it back to your literature review and clinical experiences. Once you have analyzed your data, you can then think about what the results of your analysis mean and whether there are implications for future practice.

Details of the final part of the analysis stage are not required for writing your protocol but are an important part of your preliminary planning. Thinking about what different results could tell you about your research question closes the circle and helps you assess whether or not you have worked out a logical process, whereby your initial question will be answered. To help you think about this stage we indicate some of the tasks you will eventually complete.

Actions

Immerse yourself in your data. Although this phase is usually associated with qualitative analysis it reflects the level of familiarity you need with any sort of data to ensure that your results and conclusions are rooted in your data. Here are some of the things you can do to achieve this deeper familiarity:

- Look at individual cases to understand what has happened for the individual participants over the course of your study.

- If you have qualitative data you could re-examine your transcripts and descriptive codes and make sure they relate to each other. Then look at these in relation to your analytic codes to ensure that you can track how your analysis developed from the original transcripts. You will have documented the process that you've used; now see if you can capture it in a table or diagram so that you summarize your analysis and results.

- With quantitative data, you could track through individual participant results on several assessments and make notes on their individual performances and see how these compare with your group data.

- Consider whether your results make sense to you in the light of your knowledge and what you have learned about the participants in the process of your study. Mistakes can occur with data input and any surprises need to be checked to ensure that accuracy was maintained. The opposite can also happen when we are too focused on our own expectations and have a limited view of what our data are telling us.

You will need to keep going back to your research question: remind yourself about what you are trying to find out. Data can be fascinating and we can be tempted into fishing exercises, but you need to stick to what you originally intended and wrote in your protocol. The process of conducting even small-scale studies will progress your knowledge and your thinking, but you must stick with the protocol you developed.

You will need to give yourself time for the interpretation of results. It is an exciting process that involves making that step from looking at charts, graphs, lists of themes, etc. and working out what it means. There may be an obvious short answer, but we must interrogate our data to see if that is all it is telling us and we must do this without falling prey to making unreasonable claims.

Make sure you consider your findings in the light of the strengths and weaknesses of your study. Maybe your sample size was smaller than you planned or perhaps you have reservations about one of your measures. Make sure you adjust your interpretation of your findings to take account of these strengths and limitations.

Here are a few final but important things to bear in mind with your analysis:

- Consider your results in relation to previously-published research. Are they in accord with previous trends or do they suggest there could be an alternative process at work or a different way of looking at things?

- If you are using mixed methods make sure you integrate your different findings. Your results considered in combination could tell you more than when each type of data analysis is considered independently.

- Think carefully if there are implications for future practice that you can draw from your study.

- Finally, you are in a position to review your study. What are the strengths and limitations of what you have done? Can you draw implications for future research? If you have enjoyed the process how would you like to progress your work?

8. Protocol

Purpose: to develop a protocol that will guide your investigation and inform colleagues or reviewers or governance processes about your investigation.

If you have worked through all the stages in the preceding sections then you are ready to start your practice-based evidence project – well, almost! The final step in the process is to produce a protocol. This acts as your guide and rule book for how you will carry out your project. It can act as a reminder to some of the decisions you have taken along the way and can help to make sure that you are consistent in how you collect your evidence. Being systematic in your approach is fundamental to collecting reliable evidence and a clear protocol will help you achieve that consistency. If your project involves several people, then having a clear protocol will help to ensure consistency and reliability across those working on the project. Writing the protocol is the easy bit because by now, you have done all the hard thinking, discussing and planning and you have merely to capture it on paper. The previous sections become the sections in your protocol. Below, we have set out the basic format showing how each of the headings for your protocol relate to the work you have already carried out in the previous sections.

Title

Thinking of a title for your project provides you with an easy way to refer to it; it gives it a recognizable identity that helps to remind other people, including your colleagues and participants, about what you are doing. So choose a title that gives a flavour of the project and gives the project a distinctive name. Check around on the web to make sure you are not duplicating an existing project name.

Background

This provides a summary of your initial thinking about your clinical context alongside your literature review. It should provide a justification for the project that says why it is important (to your clients or the service) and why it is needed (in terms of the gap in your existing evidence). Use the work from Steps 1 and 2 to write this section.

Question

This can be phrased in terms of your overall aims and objectives or your specific questions (Step 3).

Method and design

In this section it is useful to state your overall methods strategy and then give some particular information about your design. For example, you might say that it will be qualitative using a series of focus groups; or that it will be quantitative using a single case series; or that it will be descriptive using an audit of your caseload (Step 4).

Data collection

This will include:

- details of any participants and how you will select and recruit them to your project;
- any measures you intend to use, or the processes by which you will gather your data;
- the timing of your data collection and who will carry it out; and
- how you will manage your data and keep it confidential (Steps 5 and 6).

Analysis

You should set out how you plan to analyze your information (Step 7). This keeps you on target later when you might be tempted to keep fishing for answers beyond the original question. Sticking to your original protocol keeps the study safe in terms of your ethics and the purposes to which your participants consented and in terms of the robustness of your study.

Dissemination and reporting

An additional stage that is covered in the protocol is your plan for what you will do with your findings at the end of your project (see Chapter 9 for more information on 'Sharing your findings'). Your first responsibility is to feed back to your participants and to other people involved in your project (such as colleagues or others who helped to carry out the project). This can be a useful stage prior to more widespread dissemination as their comments and questions will help to shape the final presentation of your findings. Beyond that, it is useful to consider all the people who will want to know about your findings or people who you can influence with them. This might include your colleagues and collaborators, the local health board or commissioners. In this section of your protocol, set out all the audiences you plan to reach and show the mechanism by which you will target them, through seminars, conference presentations or workshops, through articles in public and professional magazines and in peer reviewed journals.

Project milestones

Finally, you need to think through the timescale of your project and identify key milestones. These can then help you to keep your project on track, identify any slippage and to solve problems as you go along. It is also important for your participants and other stakeholders to have some idea about the overall length of the project and when they are likely to get feedback or hear about your findings. Chapter 3 gives advice about how to keep to time scales.

Risk assessment

It is useful to read back over your protocol and think about anything that could go wrong and the possible problems that you may encounter. Think of these risks very broadly – the risks to your employing authority, to individual researchers or participants, risks regarding recruitment, timing, getting hold of resources. For each problem, try to identify in advance an alternative way to tackle that particular aspect of your project.

Summary

This chapter has provided a template for planning your piece of practice-based evidence. It indicates the questions that can guide you through the components of a sound investigation and takes the reader through the steps required to help a study run smoothly. In addition, it shows when to share your ideas with colleagues and service users so they can help you develop a workable protocol. Remember, developing a protocol is a learning experience: be prepared for setbacks and the need to rethink some stages; think about how to make best use of the resources available to you.

References

Braun, V. & Clark, V. (2006) Using thematic analysis in psychology. *Qualitative Research in Psychology*. **3:2**, 77–101.

Bryman, A. (2008) *Social Research Methods* (3rd edition). Oxford: Oxford University Press.

Glogowska, M. (2011) Paradigms, pragmatism and possibilities: Mixed methods research in speech and language therapy. *International Journal of Language and Communication Disorders* **46:3**, 251–260.

Guion, L. Diehl, D. C. and McDonald, D. (2011) *Conducting an In-depth Interview*. Institute of Food and Agricultural Sciences, University of Florida. Downloaded on 1/12/2011from edis.ifas.ufl.edu/fy393.

Kvale, S. (1996) *InterViews: An Introduction to Qualitative Research Interviewing*. Thousand Oaks, California: Sage Publications.

McCauley. R. J. & Fey, M. E. (2006) Treatment of language disorders in children. In R. J. McCauley and M. E. Fey (Eds) *Treatment of Language Disorders in Children*. Baltimore: Paul Brookes Publishing, pp. 1–17.

Merrick, R. (2011). Ethics, consent and assent when listening to children with speech, language and communication needs. In S. Roulstone & S. McLeod (Eds) *Listening to Children and Young People with Speech, Language and Communication Needs*. Guildford: J&R Press, pp. 63–72.

Medical Research Council (2008) *Developing and Evaluating Complex Interventions: New Guidance*. http://www.mrc.ac.uk/complexinterventionsguidance (issued 29 September 2008, 1st accessed January 2009).

Roulstone, S. & McLeod, S. (2011) *Listening to Children and Young People with Speech, Language and Communication Needs*. Guildford: J&R Press.

Turner, D. W. (2010) Qualitative interview design: A practical guide for novice investigators. *The Qualitative Report* Volume 15 Number 3 May 2010 754-760, available from http://www.nova.edu/ssss/QR/QR15-3/qid.pdf

Further reading

Kitzinger, J. (1995) Qualitative research: Introducing focus groups. *British Medical Journal.* **311**, 299.

Local Government Data Unit. *Wales Questionnaire Design.* Downloaded on 1 December 2011 from www.dataunitwales.gov.uk/.../CPS15010_Questionnaire_Design_FIN

Silverman, D. (2009). *Doing Qualitative Research: A Practical Handbook* (3rd Edition). London: Sage Publications.

Willig, C. (2008) *Introducing Qualitative Research in Psychology: Adventures in Theory and Method* (2nd edition). Maidenhead: Open University Press.

Resources

Resources to aid literature reviewing:
American Speech & Hearing Association: has a section on evidence-based practice which includes a compendium of evidence: http://www.asha.org/Members/ebp/default/_

SpeechBITE: An Australian-based searchable database of literature: http://www.speechbite.com/

The What Works Clearinghouse (WWC) was created in 2002 as an initiative of the U.S. Department of Education's Institute of Education Sciences (IES), to be a central and trusted source of scientific evidence for what works in education. http://ies.ed.gov/ncee/wwc/

Sites for systematic reviewing including the Cochrane Library and the Campbell Collaboration and the Evidence for Policy and Practice Information and Co-ordinating Centre (EPPI-Centre): each contain searchable databases of systematic reviews: http://www.thecochranelibrary.com/view/0/index.html

http://www.campbellcollaboration.org/

http://eppi.ioe.ac.uk/cms/

Other resources:
Centre for Evidence-Based Medicine: http://www.cebm.net/ at the University of Oxford aims to develop, teach and promote evidence-based health care and provide support and resources. Asking Focused Questions: http://www.cebm.net/?o=1036

Computer Assisted Qualitative Data AnalysiS networking Project (CAQDAS) provides support, training and other resources http://www.surrey.ac.uk/sociology/research/researchcentres/caqdas/

INVOLVE is a national advisory group that supports greater public involvement in NHS, public health and social care research. INVOLVE is funded by and is part of the National Institute of Health Research (NIHR): http://www.invo.org.uk

National Research Ethics Service (NRES): http://www.nres.nhs.uk/

3 Practicalities

Helen Stringer

Learning outcomes

By the end of this chapter, you will be able to:

- Get support from other people, both within and outside your organization
- Effectively plan time while conducting research in the context of clinical practice
- Find and appraise literature
- Know you have succeeded

Introduction

Reflection on our clinical practice is an essential part of our professional development as speech and language therapists. Being a reflective practitioner ensures that we maintain a high standard of clinical competence and that our clients get the best available service. However, it also causes us to consider the fine detail of our practice, raising issues that discussion with colleagues, supervisors and mentors often cannot resolve. Over time, the issues that arise in our practice and refuse to go away, develop into clinical questions we cannot easily find the answer to. Those burning questions are the spark to our enquiry, lighting the path to research and it is important to reignite that spark at different points along the way to remind ourselves why we are taking this journey.

No one can pretend that undertaking service evaluation or research as a practising speech and language therapist is an easy task. The very title of this book acknowledges that we are fitting research into almost non-existent gaps in our working day. However, there are many things you can do to make it possible, manageable, enjoyable and rewarding. Chapter 2 has covered the research process from turning good ideas into research questions to developing your research protocol. This chapter takes you through the process with practical ways to help it go smoothly. Aspects of the research process relating to specific types of enquiry are covered in more depth in later chapters so that whether you read from cover to cover, or dip in and out, you will be well prepared.

This chapter discusses how to search for and appraise existing literature related to your area of interest, to ensure that your question has not already been answered, either thoroughly and robustly or in a way that leaves you questioning the validity of the answer. It gives guidance to help you gain the practical support from other people that you will need at different stages of your project, ranging from your line manager and clinical colleagues to the Research and Development (R&D) department in your organization. It covers how to manage your time realistically and keep track of what you are doing, through making a Gantt chart. In addition, it suggests ways of dealing with setbacks and of recognizing the progress you are making.

Before you start

Motivation and making mates

The very fact that you have this book in your hand indicates that you have a good level of motivation for research. Sometimes, it can feel like an uphill battle, so you do need to revisit your initial enthusiasm every now and then (see below for how a research journal can become your new best friend!).

There are two types of 'motivational mates' you need to make at this stage. First, it is important to talk about your ideas and plans with a trusted colleague who is interested and can continue to share your enthusiasm as you progress. Having an interested friend can be a low-pressure way of ensuring your success. In addition, you will also need wider support. It is important to establish your research as a group endeavour with your colleagues so that you will have people to help out and support you at different stages of your project.

For example, a well organized journal club can help you with your literature review. The papers from your literature search can be critically appraised by members, spreading the workload so that it is manageable for everyone. You also have an instant discussion group, with the benefit of views from colleagues with different interests, knowledge and experience. If you do not have access to a journal club, you could have the opportunity to start one up. The benefits to a service of having a regular forum for evaluating and discussing the evidence base, while providing in-house continuing professional development (CPD) are easily sold to a manager. Although critical appraisal skills are essential, these can be picked up fairly quickly and then practised and developed in the journal club (Dollaghan, 2007; Stringer, 2010a). The next step is to organize it so that there is minimal extra work for members; for example, establish a rotation of one person per meeting to present an appraisal and lead a discussion of a paper that everyone has read. The more usual alternative to this group approach is to read and appraise the evidence base yourself. This requires good time management, discipline and good record keeping. It is essential to make notes to accompany your reading so that you only have to do it once, can quickly access the useful papers and discard the ones that you will not use again.

Colleagues can also help you out at later stages: when you need an assessor who is blind to your intervention groups, or someone to help proofread your report or journal paper when you have finished your project, or even just to return books to a library that is on their way home and not yours. Make it clear to your colleagues that these are things they can get involved in as time goes on. The advantage to them is that it helps to develop and practise their own research skills, thus raising the level of research participation in your service. Sharing skills and knowledge in this way can be a huge boost to your confidence and motivation, as you are able to tangibly track the progress you have made.

Organizational and external support

Getting the support of your manager is essential. They are ultimately responsible for what you do and will have to approve the time you spend on your project, justifying the need for it to someone higher up in the organization who might have no knowledge of your clinical area. Your manager will also have to demonstrate support if you need to go through approval processes such as R&D or ethics. In most circumstances, your manager can help you access resources, ranging from supporting the establishment of a journal club to pointing you in the direction of people with the skills you need. However, you might need to support your manager in developing the argument for research by providing a strong case for the benefits to the service and clients/service users.

Speech and language therapists (SLTs) generally have a research component written into their job descriptions, with the level of expected engagement reflecting the level of progression in our career. However, this can often be ambiguous and you may find those in more senior positions lack the research skills you already have yourself. If you want to be more research-active, the process of supervision and personal development allied to the Knowledge and Skills Framework (KSF) is the accepted route to alert your manager and to gain their support. A good manager should look out for opportunities for you once they know this is the route you wish to follow.

Discussing your research ideas with your manager at an early stage can be a time saver too. You will get more organizational support if your project contributes to their strategic plan. Your manager should be able to help you to develop a more strategic question and save you time in exploring ideas that would not be feasible to follow to completion. For example, if you are interested in interventions for dysfluency and commissioners have expressed interest in funding a new service for adolescents with dysfluency, you are more likely to get support if you tweak your plan to evaluate the effectiveness of different interventions for adolescents with dysfluent speech than if you doggedly pursue your original idea of intervention with six-year-olds.

The people in your R&D department are also helpful allies. Find out if there is an organizational research strategy and familiarize yourself with it so that you can begin to think within this framework. Organizations are generally keen to attract external funding for research projects and there might be sources of internal funding to support you in writing a large grant application. For example, in UK organizations that have already received funding from the National Institute for Health Research (NIHR), Research Capability Funding (RCF) is available and all staff are eligible to apply for it. Some organizations have well structured, supported routes for research activity. The R&D department can often put you in touch with an individual who is expert in defining research questions and developing protocols; another who is expert at data analysis (statistics) and someone else who can support you in disseminating your findings. Get to know these people before you need to draw on their support so that when the time comes you can give them exactly the information they need.

Universities can also be a good source of support for clinical researchers. You can bring knowledge and expertise in your clinical area while the academic can contribute research and academic knowledge to the partnership. If you wish to go further with your research ideas you might need to have a partnership with an academic department in order to apply for some of the available funding streams. An academic partner can support you in writing a clear and well-planned grant application, however large or small the sum of money. If you already have a relationship with a local university because you take their students on placement, you may be able to build on that and develop a research relationship.

Some universities have specific routes for clinicians to engage in research. For example, Newcastle University (UK) supports SLTs to carry out audit and small scale service evaluation through specialist student placements (Whitworth, Haining, & Stringer, 2012). Indeed, SLTs who want to engage in research are welcomed as research partners. Moreover, a collaboration of SLT Managers and academic SLTs alongside a research special interest group (SIG) provides training, support and minor funding for research projects proposed and developed by SLTs with an academic partner.

Your research journal

A research journal (or log) is an essential companion for a researcher, particularly if you are fitting research into your work and balancing clinical and research decisions and procedures. Physically, the journal can be a notebook or a document on your computer, whatever you are most comfortable with.

You will use your research journal every time you work on your project, from the very early stages until you have finished. If you have a meeting about your project with anyone, it is good practice to email them with a summary of the content and outcome of the meeting, giving them the opportunity to add their own perceptions. Record the date of the meeting in your journal, along with a link to or copy of emails. This is particularly helpful if, for example, your manager changes and you need to bring the new manager up to speed with commitments the organization has made to you.

Throughout the process of your research project you will be making decisions where you weigh up several alternatives and decide to go for one and not the others, such as, for example, deciding to classify articulation errors as correct phonemes, but devoicing as a phonological error. It is essential that you record these decisions together with your rationale, because on another day, talking with another person, you might make a different, equally valid decision. The consequence of losing track of your decision-making processes is that you can end up with methodological inconsistencies that can affect the progress of your project and its success.

The contents of your journal will be invaluable when it comes to writing up your project, making the process quicker and more reliable. It is also a good way of reminding yourself how much you have learned and achieved when you go to your next supervision or appraisal meeting.

Patient and Public Involvement (PPI)

This topic is addressed throughout this book. Just to note here that it is vital to involve service users and/or members of the public in the planning of your research. This can be on any level, from a formal user group that discusses the benefits and outcomes of research in relation to their needs, to a few parents in the waiting room who you ask informally to look over a draft of your information booklet. Draw up a PPI strategy and timetable at an early stage in your planning so that you are not held up by unexpected logistical issues such as difficulties booking a suitable meeting room. There are established service user groups in many clinical areas that are often willing to support research development. Social networks can be useful in finding interested people and you may find that setting up a Facebook Group or starting a Twitter hashtag (#) quickly generates a group of people who can help with your PPI plans in some way. However, be aware of the limitations and regulations of your employing institution with regard to use of the internet.

Getting started

Search for and appraise relevant literature

Time is a precious and expensive commodity. It is essential that we don't waste it pursuing questions that have already been answered. The time you spend looking for existing research and critically appraising it is time very well spent.

As an SLT working in the UK you have many options for accessing literature. Information about papers in all academic journals is now held on web-based databases, so access to the internet is crucial. NHS employees have access to the NHS online library and to local NHS libraries, often housed in the education department of a hospital. In addition, university libraries usually have membership categories for NHS staff and others who will benefit from using the library; it is well worth exploring membership either online or by phone. If either of those two resources is impractical or unavailable, you will be able to make use of your local public library membership. Whichever library you are using, get to know your librarian and the specialist skills they have (Stringer, 2010b). Your librarian can teach you how to do effective database searches and might often do them for you. Although some databases, e.g. Google Scholar or PubMed, are freely available (open access), some are only available through library subscription, requiring an Athens password (e.g. Web of Knowledge, Ovid).

Databases are selective search engines that automatically limit the results of a search to items that have particular relevance for your search terms. For example, if you type 'LSVT' into Google, you will get over 42,000 results, not all of them relating to the Lee Silverman Voice Treatment (LSVT®). Google is a general search engine and looks for results all over the internet. If you type 'LSVT' into Google Scholar, which only searches 'scholarly literature', you will get about 1700 results, all related to the intervention. The more selective databases that require an Athens (or Shibboleth) password will return even fewer results because they are even more selective of the journals they search. Using LSVT® as an example: Web of Knowledge (covering sciences, social sciences, arts and humanities) returned 120 results; Ovid returned 239, which reduced to 141 once duplicates were removed; ERIC is an education database which returned just seven results. Ovid is a major database platform that includes a wide range of separate databases, all accessed through one search page. You choose which databases you search and can even specify the dates, e.g. after 2008, so this is a very efficient way of searching a wide range of journals. Ovid includes Medline (health sciences, also freely available as PubMed), PsychInfo (psychology) and EBM (Evidence Based Medicine) reviews (including the Cochrane reviews). Most databases will allow you to save your search, if you create an account, which usually just involves giving your email address and a password. They also export the references to reference management software such as EndNote, ProCite, RefWorks, Mendeley, Zotero (the last two are freely available to download). The software stores your references and most also interface with word processing programs to insert citations and create reference lists in your paper as you write it, taking seconds rather than the hours it would take to do that manually. As mentioned above, your librarian can help you make sense of the databases and reference management; starting off with a training session, however brief, will increase your efficiency.

Use your research journal to record exactly what you searched for and what you found. This should include: your search terms; the databases you searched; how many papers turned up on each search; how many are relevant (what criteria you used to decide this); and how many you can access as full versions. This will save you a lot of time when you come to do another search, by preventing unnecessary duplication; it is remarkably hard to remember the exact search terms from your first search by the time you are on your fourth.

Abstracts of papers are widely available with open access, but full versions of papers are often only available by subscription or through inter-library loans (ILL). It could be worth asking your manager to set up an account with your organization library to cover the cost of ILL so that you and your colleagues can easily access papers if they are not available online. You can read the abstract to get an idea of how relevant the paper is to your question but information in an abstract might be inconsistent with or absent from the main body of the paper (Pitkin, Branagan, & Burmeister, 1999). Only the full version of the paper will tell you what really happened.

It is not possible to predict how many papers your literature search will come up with. It could be one or two, which are easy to deal with, but it could be a much larger number. Once you have sifted through the abstracts and decided which papers are really relevant (e.g. is it about the same client group, intervention or outcome?), it is time to read them. Embarking on your own research project, you are now a peer of the researcher who wrote the paper. You may feel a long way from them in terms of experience, but remember that they will also have made the same first steps as you.

Critical appraisal is an essential skill when you are evaluating existing evidence and thinking about your own research question. You must remain objective and, on occasion, set aside your beliefs about the work you do. For instance, if you have used one particular assessment for a long time it could be challenging to read a paper that clearly demonstrates that a different assessment is more reliable and accurate; but your commitment to quality will allow you to step outside your comfort zone and critically appraise the new evidence, potentially leading you to change a long-established practice and challenging your beliefs about it.

There are resources and courses available to support your development of critical appraisal skills. Starting with the internet, for example, resources are available on the Royal College of Speech and Language Therapists' website and from the Centre for Evidence Based Medicine (see Resources at the end of this chapter). Training in critical appraisal skills is also available through NHS organizations or can be organized through clinical network and special interest groups.

It is important to record the outcome of your critical appraisal of a paper in a consistent and practical way. There are many critical appraisal checklists available online, for example at the Critical Appraisal Skills Programme (CASP) website and the Scottish Inter-collegiate Network (SIGN) website and in books (see Greenhalgh, 2010).

You may prefer to design your own checklist, possibly with a colleague. Table 3.1 provides an example of a checklist with headings to evaluate quality and to identify aspects of the paper that could eventually be used in a funding application or discussion of a paper. You can make your own checklist to suit the type of project you are doing and adjust the questions accordingly.

Be thorough in your literature search and celebrate if you find a comprehensive and thorough evidence-based answer to your question. You can then move on to another idea you have been nurturing.

Table 3.1 A critical appraisal checklist designed specifically for collecting information to support an intervention study.

Nicholson-Stringer Critical Appraisal Tool for literature reviews	
Title	
Year	
Authors	
Journal	
Introduction/background Useful references and interesting points	
Research questions	
Hypothesis	
Method	
Participants Selection criteria Inclusion/exclusion Age Gender Socio-Economic Status data Bias?	

(cont. overleaf)

Methodology	
Procedure	
Clearly described	
Replicable	
Frequency	
Delivered by?	
Timing	
Treatment fidelity	
Blinding	
Bias	
Follow up	
Measures	
What are they?	
Do they measure what they say they do?	
Standardized/published	
Reliable etc?	
When?	
Outcomes	
Primary outcome stated?	
Secondary outcomes?	
Proposed analysis	
What tests are proposed?	
Results	
Analysis	
Did they do what they said they would?	
Post hoc analysis	
Data omissions?	
Have data been omitted?	
How are missing data are accounted for?	

(cont.)

Findings Significant/non-significant? Effect sizes?	
Anomalies Effect of variables not accounted for Selection bias Maturational effects External effects	
Attrition	
Follow up	
Discussion	
Are research questions answered?	
Are effects accurately reported? Or overstated?	
Weaknesses acknowledged?	
Explanation Theory Relation to existing literature Is it plausible?	
Implications For future research For clinical practice	
Further comments	

Time management

As has been mentioned in Chapter 2, the end result of your planning will be a protocol that will guide you when conducting your research. When writing your protocol you need to assign tasks to a timeline to show how the project tasks will progress, and provide a start and end date. You will be asked for this information by your R&D department and ethics committee if you need approvals (see below for help with the processes involved here).

The accepted way to present this is in a Gantt chart. A Gantt chart is essentially a calendar of the tasks you have to perform to complete your research. The internet is your best source of information here. If you Google 'Gantt chart' you will get over 3 million results, but the first few are likely to be the most informative. Look at Gantt charts for a variety of different types of project and you will get a good idea of the level of detail needed and how you can keep a hold of the detail of your project (see 'getting into the detail' in subsequent chapters).

You can use specialist software to draw up your Gantt chart, or commonly-used programs such as Excel or Word. Essentially, you are creating a table that lists every task in your project against the timeline you have decided upon. See Table 3.2 for an example of a Gantt chart for a project to evaluate SLT interventions over a 16-month timeline.

When estimating how much time you will take to complete a task, remember that you are probably also working and carrying out your everyday activities, so be realistic with regard to how much you can achieve in the time you have. It is often said that you should multiply any estimate of time by three to get the real idea of how long a task will take. However, you will know from the way you manage time in your work that you are more efficient at some tasks than others. Use that knowledge when drawing up your Gantt chart. Make sure you add in your annual leave and any other things that routinely impact on life such as public or school holidays. Also think about things that impact on your potential participants that might affect your time management; for example, if your older participants look after grandchildren it may restrict their availability, or if you live in a place where public transport is disrupted every winter due to bad weather your participants might not be able to come to their therapy sessions. It is advisable to add in an extra few weeks to cover these eventualities and allow for catch-up sessions. It is much harder to find extra time during your project than to add it in the planning stage. A good tip is to work backwards from your end date and divide up the time according to the various tasks that need to be done.

Approval processes

In Chapter 1 you read about the difference between audit, service evaluation and research. Your R&D department will only be involved in research but they have useful information that can help you with audit and service evaluation, such as gaining consent, producing information sheets, etc. The process for

Table 3.2 An example of a Gantt chart for a project to evaluate SLT interventions over a 16-month timeline.

Year												1				2
Month	1	2	3	4	5	6	7	8	9	10	11	12	13	14	15	16
Ethics application	▒	▒	▒													
Recruitment of RA		▒	▒	▒												
Complete manuals for interventions	▒	▒	▒	▒												
Develop intervention resources	▒	▒	▒	▒												
Recruit 20 participants			▒													
Assessment 1			▒													
Intervention					▒	▒	▒	▒	▒	▒	▒					
Assessment 2					▒											
Treatment fidelity check							▒	▒								
Survey of parents and teachers						▒										
Follow up Assessment 3										▒						
Data analysis				▒									▒	▒	▒	
Steering group meeting				▒							▒					
Preparing peer-reviewed papers														▒	▒	▒
Dissemination of findings														▒	▒	▒

NHS R&D approval for research can be long, complex and frustrating. R&D governance and ethical approval are in place to ensure that both participants and researchers are safe and only exposed to the minimum amount of considered risk. Having this in mind will help you approach both these processes with an appropriate attitude.

If you work in the NHS, or want to include NHS staff or patients/service users in your research, you will be required to adhere to the Research Governance structure/framework. The best place to find the most up-to-date version of this is on the UK Department of Health website. Check for different versions for the devolved countries. Even if you do not work in the NHS, it is worth reading this document, as it gives a good idea of the issues that arise when planning research and the type of risks and other issues relating to research and good clinical practice that should be addressed.

As soon as you are at the point of knowing you have a question to answer and have agreement from your manager, contact the R&D department and arrange to talk to someone about the process, get copies of any paperwork you need and deadlines for completion. If they understand your project from the beginning they can give you more appropriate support and help the process go more smoothly and quickly. Remember that they are likely to deal with many more projects involving invasive procedures such as drug trials, than behavioural procedures such as SLT interventions. You might have to do a lot of information sharing so that the R&D department has a good understanding of, for example, the level of risk to your participants, the status of your manager compared to a medical consultant, and issues related to sponsorship and insurance. Research projects need to have indemnity insurance, unlike service evaluation or audit which are covered by the insurance for your usual practice. The R&D department usually covers this automatically when it signs off the permission, but arrangements for this vary from one organization to another so raise it at an early stage in your discussions. R&D departments are increasingly requiring researchers to attend specific training courses before projects are given approval; these could include Good Clinical Practice and Informed Consent. Once again, check at the very beginning of your planning as the courses are usually in great demand and you might have to book several months ahead. If you are planning a research project with participants identified through the NHS you also need ethical approval.

All research projects require ethical approval, but systems for approval differ depending upon who is participating in the research. If the participants are recruited outside the NHS there might not be an ethical approval process in place. If you are planning on recruiting school students or residents in a care home, you need to check with the Local Authority what ethical approvals have to be obtained before your research can be carried out. If there is no formal ethical approval in place it is absolutely your responsibility to ensure that any ethical issues have been suitably addressed. For guidance on this and information regarding whether or not you need NHS ethics approval, always check with your R&D department before embarking on any research activity.

If you are recruiting participants who are being identified because they are NHS patients, for example clients on your caseload, patients attending a particular clinic or with a particular diagnosis, then you will have to obtain NHS ethical approval. The NHS process for ethical approval is constantly evolving and being refined in response to feedback from users. It is currently a time-sensitive online process, and is accessed through the Integrated Research Application System (IRAS, see www.myreserachproject.org.uk). This system integrates both R&D and ethical approvals, minimizing the repetition of information that needs to be entered. There is a lot of helpful information, example forms and e-learning on this website and you do not have to work for the NHS to access it. You will need to have your research protocol and be able to describe your project in terms that a lay person can understand. Try talking it through first with someone very removed from what you do. You cannot just copy and paste from your protocol. Take this as a good opportunity to go through your project in minute detail and visualize how it will work in practice. You might find that you go back to your protocol and do some tweaking at this stage.

Data storage and security is scrutinized by the ethics committee (see below). The committee might encourage you to store your data for a longer time so that you can get maximum benefit from it, for example, by doing secondary analysis or analyzing an aspect of the data not included in your original plan. Storage of data should comply with the Data Protection Act (1998) which states that data for research purposes can be stored indefinitely only if the data are useful and relevant. The ethics committee will give you guidance on this matter, including on issues such as how to word information and consent to include storage and future use of data.

You will also have to describe how you will maintain the anonymity of your participants. The traditional way of doing this is to allocate the participants an identification (ID) code and have the key to that code, i.e. the list of names and corresponding confidential identifiers, locked in a filing cabinet to which only the lead researchers have access. Using a password-protected electronic document is the 21st century version of that process.

Along with your R&D and ethical approval forms you will have to submit for approval all the other paperwork that goes with your project. This includes test protocols and assessment record forms as well as the information and consent leaflets you will use. Sample information and consent forms are available from the IRAS website. However, these are intended for participants who do not have communication disorders. You will have to make sure your information and consent forms can be understood by your participants. This could mean writing them in simple, accessible language; using illustrations; making an interactive video that can be viewed on a laptop or television; providing translated versions, etc. I always bind my information sheets in an A5 booklet with a question-and-answer format. It is really helpful at this stage to ask a group of service users if they find your information sheets and consent forms easy to follow. If you are aiming to recruit children you will need information for them as well as the person who has parental responsibility. You will need to find out who is legally responsible for giving consent, for example, the person who has parental responsibility for a child; or in some psychiatric facilities it might be the psychiatrist in charge who gives consent, not the patient.

Recruiting participants

In a small-scale service evaluation it is likely that you will be recruiting participants from your own caseload or in collaboration with colleagues. You will have to ensure that your recruitment strategy does not coerce the participant in any way and demonstrate that as part of the ethical process. If you are relying on other people to recruit participants for you it is worth thinking about what would encourage them to do this. For example, is there a benefit to their service? Do they have a vested interest in the potential benefit to the participant? Spend some time discussing your project with them and make sure you both understand what the issues around recruitment are. Remember to send that confirmation email so you both have in writing what you discussed and agreed. It is important to bear in mind that, if recruiting through the NHS, invitations to participants must come from a source known to them, for example, their SLT.

Dealing with data

As you progress with your project and collect data, make sure you are storing it in a way that will be useful when it comes to later analysis. You might want to use a spreadsheet format such as Excel rather than a table in a document. Data in a spreadsheet can be organized, filtered and searched; you can perform basic statistics on it and make charts and graphs. It is easy to add in new columns and you can use different pages without needing to create a new document, so that all of your data are in one place. You can also easily transfer it into statistical software. When storing data on a computer, think carefully how you will label and date your documents and files so that you know what is in them and which one is the most current. It is probably worth dedicating a page in your research journal to file names and document versions.

Remember that, in whatever format it is in, all data should be securely kept, so encryption, passwords and locked cabinets are in order. Talk to your local IT support to find out about the latest in document security, as this is an area that develops rapidly and the method you use will depend on the operating system on your computer and the software you use. You will need a locked filing cabinet or cupboard to store any paper records and data, for example the record sheets and consent forms. You will need secure space on your computer hard drive or server for your electronic data. You may need to negotiate extra server space with your IT department.

You will also need a reliable and secure back-up process. Ideally, this is provided by the organization you work for, on secure remote servers. Many organizations, including the NHS, do not permit staff to use any other form of data storage. If that facility is not available to you, if you accidentally delete data, or get a virus, or your computer crashes, you can sometimes find an expert who can retrieve it for you, but there may be no means of recovering it and no way to collect it again. At the very least, you should back-up your data onto an external hard drive every day and lock it up with your consent forms. Personally (and learned from bitter experience), I back up data onto a portable hard drive every time I change them, for example, every time I enter new data, so that I have a snap shot. If you are applying for external funding for your research it is reasonable to request funding for secure data storage, particularly if you are storing large audio and video files. Secure data storage is something that you will have to detail in applying for any approvals you require.

As you go along

Support and mentoring

It is a good idea to have a page in your research journal that documents what support and mentoring you thought you needed when you started planning your research. Revisit that when you are in the middle of collecting your data and reflect on your current needs and make sure they are being fulfilled. Do you need to schedule an update meeting with your manager, or do you need a coffee with your motivating friend? If you need a meeting with the statistician in three weeks' time, do you know what format they want your data in and do you know if they have time in their diary to see you?

Making progress

As SLTs we are skilled at planning interventions that have built-in flexibility so that they are responsive to our clients' needs. During a session, we will quickly change a line of discussion, make an activity harder or easier, cut something short or make something longer. Put simply, we are very good at thinking on our feet and solving potential problems before they arise. That skill is immediately transferable to your research project. Inevitably it will not go exactly as you planned; there are too many variables for everything to be utterly predictable. The main thing to do when things are apparently going awry is to keep calm and keep your sense of humour.

Keep your Gantt chart at hand so that you can regularly check your progress against your plan. It is easier to deal with time slippage of a few days than a few months. Write deadlines in your diary and put in a warning ten days before so that you can plan time to catch up if necessary. We have already mentioned the usefulness of a paper trail if your manager decides to move on to pastures new. If something happens that is likely to upset your timeline significantly, for example, recruitment is slower than you expected, or you get the 'flu and have an unexpected week off, deal with it calmly and renegotiate the timing with your manager and others involved in the project. If the consultant recruiting your participants goes on maternity leave, ask her to identify the person who will pick up that role and join you in a meeting to gain that person's cooperation. Whatever you do, don't pretend that nothing has happened and ignore it; unexpected events happen to all researchers and if you manage them efficiently and effectively it will only enhance your experience and reputation as a researcher.

If your project has a long timeline, at the 12-month point you will have to complete a progress report for the ethics committee that gave you approval. This is a good point at which to reflect on what you have achieved, as sometimes you can get lost in the process and lose sight of the amount of work you have completed.

The finishing point

Dissemination

Chapter 9 *Sharing Your Findings* gives detailed advice on writing up and other means of disseminating your findings. At this stage, you can look back through your research journal and make a list of all the people you need to inform about your project and think about the best way of doing this: for your participants this could be a personal report about their involvement; for people who helped to recruit participants it might be a summary of data for their patients; a presentation at the staff meeting for your colleagues; a report to the R&D department or a poster for the staff room of the school that helped you out.

It is wise to start writing up almost as soon as you start your project. If you have carried out research and not written it up and made it accessible in the public domain through publication then, to all intents and purposes, the research does not exist. Writing up may appear to be an add-on, but it is central to the whole research process. Your research journal will be essential in the writing-up process, as much of the detail will be there. It is usually easier to start by writing the methodology, as that is the very factual part, it is usually the quickest part to write and you can have a good sense of achievement as you go on to write the other sections. While writing up, use your colleagues and your own critical appraisal skills to keep a check on style and content.

Using your findings

Having found an answer to your question, you should consider how this will change your practice. You may also find you have developed more questions than answers! This can form the basis for further research and place you in a position to move on to the next stage.

What to do with new skills

One of the most rewarding things about completing a research project is to look back at what you were like at the beginning and compare it to where you are now. The knowledge and skills you have acquired can now be used in other research projects and other aspects of your work; see Chapter 10 *Moving On* for more information about the next steps you can take in the research side of your career. You can use some of the processes you set up to support your project to progress the development and implementation of evidence-based practice in your department. You can share your networks to support colleagues to develop their own research activity. Finally, you can enjoy the sense of achievement in so many areas and feel good about moving on to the next stage of your career.

Summary

When embarking on a study, it is important to find sources of support and help and keep a research journal. In addition, you need to establish that your research question has not already been adequately answered by someone else. Patient and Public Involvement (PPI) in research is not only valuable but also essential. You might need to gain approval from ethics and R&D, depending on your type of investigation. Planning your time effectively will help you keep on track. Data storage and handling needs careful consideration. Your findings will hopefully inform your practice which you should share with others through dissemination.

References

Dollaghan, C. (2007) *The Handbook for Evidence-Based Practice in Communication Disorders.* Baltimore: Paul H Brookes Publishing Co.

Greenhalgh, T. (2010) *How to Read a Paper* (4th ed.). London: BMJ Books.

Pitkin, R. M., Branagan, M. A., & Burmeister, L. F. (1999) Accuracy of data in abstracts of published research articles. *Journal of the American Medical Association* **281:12** 1110–1111.

Stringer, H. (2010a). Evaluating the written evidence. *RCSLT Bulletin*, October, 22.

Stringer, H. (2010b) Searching for evidence. *RCSLT Bulletin*, September, 22.

Whitworth, A., Haining, S., & Stringer, H. (2012) Enhancing research capacity across healthcare and higher education sectors: Development and evaluation of an integrated model. *BMC Health Services Research* **12(1)**, 287. doi: 10.1186/1472-6963-12-287

Further reading

Body, R. & McAllister, L. (2009) *Ethics in Speech and Language Therapy*. Chichester: Wiley- Blackwell.

Crombie, I. K. (1996) *The Pocket Guide to Critical Appraisal*. London: BMJ Publishing.

Peat, J., Barton, B., & Elliott, E. (2008) *Statistics Workbook for Evidence-based Health Care*. Chichester: Wiley-Blackwell/BMJ Books.

Roddam, H., and Skeat, J. (2010) *Embedding Evidence-Based Practice in Speech and Language Therapy: International Examples*. Chichester: Wiley-Blackwell.

Stringer, H. (2010a) Formulating evidence-based practice questions. *RCSLT Bulletin*, August, 22.

Stringer, H. (2010b) What is evidence-based practice? *RCSLT Bulletin*, July, 22.

Resources

American Speech-Language Hearing Association (ASHA) has a very good research and evidence-based practice section on their website: http://www.asha.org/research/

Centre for Evidence Based Medicine website: http://www.cebm.net

Critical Appraisal Skills Programme (CASP) website: http://www.casp-uk.net

Integrated Research Application Service (IRAS) for NHS ethical approval applications: http://www.myresearchproject.org.uk/

National Institute for Health Research (NIHR) website: http://www.nihr.ac.uk

Research and Development Information (R&D Info) provides information and support for health service researchers, based in the University of Leeds: http://www.rdinfo.org.uk/

Royal College of Speech and Language Therapists' website: http://www.rcslt.org

Scottish Inter-collegiate Network (SIGN) website: http://www.sign.ac.uk

Part II How to turn clinical questions into research

4 Does my intervention make a difference to my client's impairment?

Corinne Dobinson and Nick Miller

Learning outcomes

By the end of this chapter, you will be able to:

- Refine a broad clinical query into a research question and form a hypothesis
- Have an awareness of the types of research design that might be most suitable to use to answer your question
- Give consideration to the confounding variables that could influence outcomes
- Understand validity, reliability and forms of bias

Introduction

Several of the chapters in this book are directed at helping you to gauge how your intervention affects your client. In this chapter, we focus specifically on gathering information from your everyday clinical practice about the impact your intervention has on your client's impairment. We will also help you learn how to turn this information into data that will answer questions based on your own curiosity or challenges from others, such as commissioners, managers, the research community or individual clients and their families. Since we cannot cover every issue in the chapter, we will endeavour to address those that we consider are most important and guide you in seeking further support.

Definitions

Before we go on, just a few words defining what we think lies behind the chapter title.

Impairment is the term employed in the World Health Organisation's (WHO) International Classification of Function, Disability and Health (ICF) (World Health Organisation, 2007) to signify disruption at the level of bodily structure and function (see Chapter 1 of this book, and Hartelius & Miller 2010). In the present context, therefore, this covers variables such as voice quality, rate of speech, speed and complexity of syntactic processing, minimal pair judgements, and so forth. This is in contrast to *activity* and *participation* which are also described in the ICF and are discussed in Chapter 5 of this book.

Intervention is used broadly in this chapter to mean any clinical input that might influence the impairment. Thus, questions posed could be about a specific therapy technique, or the way a therapy is delivered, for example intensive versus non-intensive or in school versus clinic environments. Alternatively, questions could relate to the timing of the therapy, such as treating immediately after stoke versus three months post onset; or about the people who are delivering the intervention, for example SLT assistants versus SLTs.

The term *make a difference* is trickier. Remaining strictly within an impairment mode one meaning might be does voice quality have less jitter and shimmer? Are the number of syllables per second in rate of speech reduced? Is upper oesophageal sphincter relaxation triggered earlier? Is word retrieval faster? One might therefore look for a statistically significant improvement in comparing assessment scores before and after intervention or in one condition versus another. However, it is important to note that a statistically significant change is not necessarily a clinically significant change. Ideally, you wish to know if the altered performance in impairment actually makes a difference to the person's ability to communicate (or swallow); indeed, you might think that the functional outcome of your intervention is of primary importance. It is therefore crucial that the measures you use to see if your intervention has made a difference reflect the changes you are trying to bring about. Accordingly, alongside measuring impairment, it will be important to describe and measure changes on other levels of functioning, including outcomes measured against what a client has defined as a key goal for him or herself. For further information on these areas, see Chapter 5 for addressing quality of life issues and Chapter 6 for gathering data on clients' and others' perspectives.

What are the issues and challenges?

Clinical issues

As we can see from Chapter 1, there are many issues relating to clinical practice that might drive you to seek an answer to the question that forms our chapter title. As competition for clinical resources increases we are constantly being challenged to provide evidence of the impact of our intervention. NHS clinicians are required to develop and evaluate innovative methods of delivering intervention that will provide quality care whilst being cost effective and efficient, and to convince commissioners to this effect.

Evidence gathering issues

In gathering evidence you will face challenges to ensure that the evidence you provide is valid and reliable and will stand up to scrutiny. By asking yourself a few questions at the outset, it is possible to develop a structure or method to support your evidence gathering to fulfil these criteria. These have been addressed generally in Chapter 2, but we will revisit them here in relation to the specific topic of this chapter and structure the forthcoming sections around them.

The first challenge for someone who wants to carry out research is to pose a clear, answerable and meaningful question. This may seem obvious, but a general clinical query can often be vague and you will need to pin it down and define precisely what it is you want to know. You need to be aware of the size of the question you are asking and whether you have the resources to answer it (time, personnel, finance, available participants, etc) or, if not, how you could obtain them. When planning the methods you are going to use to answer your question, another challenge will be deciding what measures to use to determine the outcome of your intervention. It is important that they are appropriate and provide information directly relevant to your question, but you also need to consider the burden on the clients who will become your participants. You may well find you have to make tricky decisions to arrive at an acceptable compromise between a high standard of scientific integrity and the reality of the clinical context. There might also be challenges with regard to your intervention, such as deferment of further treatment prior to a follow-up measure or more frequent visits to the clinic than would normally be expected. These issues will also be raised by your ethics committee (if you are conducting research rather than a service evaluation) whose job it is to protect participants.

In the following sections, we will present the steps that you need to take in order to answer a question related to the chapter title.

What do we already know about it?

You might not be the first to ask your question. It could be that someone has already tried to answer it. Even if not, they may have answered a similar one which could help you shape your question or the way you go about answering it. It is therefore important to conduct a literature review and appraise carefully any evidence you discover. Chapter 3 gives practical advice on doing a literature search. Here we address searching and appraising the literature with specific reference to the impact of intervention upon impairment.

Literature search

Gathering literature can be unpredictable. On occasions, you might be overwhelmed by the sheer volume. At other times, you can be surprised so little exists. By thinking carefully about how you search the literature you can save time and effort.

What types of literature should I be looking for?

When looking for literature that evaluates the impact of intervention on impairment there are several types of literature we can look for and we should include these types in our search terms.

Some papers may have already gathered the existing evidence in *meta-analyses* and *systematic reviews*. Meta-analysis is a statistical technique for combining the results of separate smaller studies to be equivalent to one larger-scale investigation. Meta-analyses are dependent upon systematic reviews.

Systematic reviews gather all relevant published research relating to a specified question. The quality of the studies is systematically appraised with reference to the methods used, how they were conducted and the validity and reliability of the outcomes. Papers are discarded if they do not fit the criteria of the review, or if the quality of the work is not deemed sufficiently high. The results of the remaining papers are then reviewed. The systematic review could be published as it stands to answer the question. Probably the best known systematic reviews in evidence-based medicine are the Cochrane reviews (see the Resources section at the end of this chapter). Several journals are devoted to providing annual reviews or current opinions in different areas.

In the field of meta-analysis and systematic reviews, as with other types of study, there are different levels of evidence. (More information about levels of evidence can be found on the websites in the resources section at the end of this chapter.) Some reviews are highly selective in what they will permit as evidence, for example, including only large scale randomized controlled trials (RCTs). Whilst drug trials are well suited to RCTs, in fields such as SLT there could be barriers to conducting such studies. Indeed, behavioural interventions on complex conditions such as those commonly used in SLT could be more suited to an alternative type of research investigation, so reviews which are limited to RCTs may conclude there is no evidence to support a particular intervention. In this case it is important to probe further and seek indications from other study types which might answer your question, such as single case designs, case series or small group studies. However, it is important to remain mindful of the nature and quality of the evidence they provide.

Whatever the level of evidence, studies reported in the literature or elsewhere can help you plan your own investigation. You will not only find out if someone has already addressed your question, but also gather information about how others undertook the work. You will be aware of the methodological issues, what was used to measure change, the obstacles that had to be overcome and how, if possible, this was achieved. Sometimes you will discover why aspects still remain unaddressed; for example, if there was difficulty finding a suitable methodology or measurement technique or there was an insufficient number of participants. In addition, although you may start by looking at studies that answer similar clinically-based research questions to your own, it could also be worthwhile spreading the net wider when you begin to think about the more detailed aspects of your study. For example, if you are having difficulty thinking of the methods you want to use, you might want to find out how this type of research question has been answered in a different population or by a different discipline.

What terms should I be using in my search?

First of all, write down the question you are asking as best you can, as the key words and phrases you have used will help you. Think of the type of evidence you are looking for: for example, *meta-analysis, systematic review, efficacy, effectiveness.* If you have a particular therapy or intervention you want to investigate, use this term also: for example, *phonological therapy, LSVT®, word-finding therapy.* Use a term that reflects the people or population for whom this intervention is relevant, for example, *stroke, Parkinson's disease, adult learning difficulties, specific language impairment.* Consider what other key words or phrases might be directly connected with your question, for example, *home practice, intensive, computer-assisted, schools, group.* You might also wish to use terms that reflect outcome, for example, *outcome, effects* (in the USA termed '*response to intervention*'), *treatment effects, improvement, deterioration, generalization.*

You will probably find that certain authors or research teams appear repeatedly in your searches. Look at the dates of their publications as these can reveal the direction and progress of their research. Work backwards from their latest reports. They may also be citing other key work in the field that you can follow up.

As you read, you may find that one particular paper, seminal text, or set of papers is constantly cited. This usually indicates the key paper or papers that underpin this theme of research and often from which other branches of research have formed. It is important you read these key papers as they will provide relevant background information for your study. However, you should still appraise them carefully, so you are aware of their limitations and understand how this influenced later studies.

Appraising the evidence

Once you have decided what you need to read, ensure that it is valid. Chapter 3 provides an appraisal checklist (see Table 3.1) which will help you do this. There are also guides on websites, details of which can be found in the further reading section of this chapter.

Refining the question

Using the information from your literature review, you are now in a position to refine your question further, making it something that is precise, answerable, manageable and workable. In relation to looking at whether your intervention changes your client's impairment, you can do this by asking:

- What, specifically, am I trying to change in terms of the *impairment*? For example, naming, auditory comprehension of sentences, phonology, attention.

- Who will be involved? For example, people with acute stroke, Parkinson's disease, pre-school children, people with dysarthria, dysphagia.

- How am I going to attempt to change it? That is, what is the intervention (describe in detail in terms of type of activity, frequency of delivery, agent providing intervention such as parent, carer or SLT, duration of intervention, etc.).

- What am I comparing? For example, before and after treatment, two different approaches, group versus individual.

- How will I compare it? For example, what scores will I compare and what statistical or other analytical method will I need?

- What do I consider is going to count as a change? For example, will it be an 8dB increase in intensity, 10% reduction in speaking rate, minimum score increase of 5/100 on a naming task?

Developing a manageable question

Ideally, you should have a simple, straightforward yes–no question. Even so, apparently simple questions can hide a host of hurdles which can trip you up even before the study starts. Like this one: is Newcastle hotter than Bristol? Straightforward enough, but which Bristol (UK, Virginia, Tennessee)? Which Newcastle (New South Wales, Tyne and Wear, Co. Down)? Once this issue is resolved, there is the problem of how do you define 'hotter'? Is it about the temperature or the social scene? How will you measure it? This is not simply a case of selecting Celsius or Fahrenheit, but key decisions such as whether to measure one specific day a year or take the mean over a whole year or decade. Should you measure just daylight temperature (and when does that start and finish?) or the 24-hour mean? Will you adjust for altitude? On the other hand, you may want to simply ask people what they think.

To start with we need to define what we mean by Newcastle, Bristol, hotter and so forth. In evidence-gathering parlance this is formulating our *operational definitions*. We also need to decide exactly how we will measure the difference in things like temperature by being aware of the *procedural issues*.

Exercise

Chapter 2 gives an exercise in refining a question; here we provide a further one, specifically in relation to our chapter title. In Table 4.1, we have provided some questions directly related to SLT clinical practice. Consider whether each question is directly answerable in its current form; if not, think about what makes it unanswerable and try to refine it so that it can be answered. Thinking back to all the issues with Newcastle versus Bristol, analyze each word in the question and decide what the operational definition will be (is one possible?) and how you will measure outcomes. Consider also what factors you need to control to get a reliable answer and, therefore, a refined question.

Table 4.1 Questions to try to refine.

- Does wearing a cueing brooch reduce drooling in people with Parkinson's disease?
- Is metrical pacing more effective than delayed auditory feedback at maintaining fluent speech in people who stutter?
- Does improving breath and phonation control in children with cerebral palsy increase their intelligibility?
- Does using an ABC chart improve intelligibility and acceptability of speech in speakers with dysarthria?
- Does regular hydration lead to better voice quality?
- Is nonverbal gestural naming significantly better than spoken naming in my client with Broca's aphasia?
- Does electrical stimulation improve swallowing transit time in people with dysphagia?
- Does the Whizzolips Programme improve intelligibility in children with phonological impairment?

Dependent and independent variables

Before we move on from question development, there are two more notions we need to consider. Firstly, in refining your question you must determine the *variables*. To do this you need to consider where you expect change to take place; for example, sound pressure level/loudness, perceived voice quality, number of semantic errors, or whatever. This is termed your *dependent variable* (often abbreviated to DV). You will wish to see if the DV is influenced by other factors or variables, for example, therapy (before versus after), speaking context (classroom versus playground; reading versus conversation). These other conditions are termed the *independent variables* (IV). If you are going to conduct your own analyses it is imperative to identify variables. When you seek support from a statistician colleague their first question is likely to be, *What are your DVs and IVs?*'

Exercise

Here are a few scenarios for practice at identifying DVs and IVs. Read the statements and identify the DV and IV in each. The answers can be found at the end of this chapter'

1. You want to compare the vocabulary skills of 8-year-olds in your language unit with 8-year-olds in the general population.

2. You want to know if a bilingual speaker is more prone to stuttering in one language than the other.

3. The effects of social skill training for a 23-year-old male with learning disability were explored. You compare amount of eye-contact during conversations before versus after your intervention.

Developing a hypothesis

When you have refined your question, you are well on your way to developing a *hypothesis*. A hypothesis is a prediction, your informed bet, of what you think the outcome of your question will be. When seeking support from a statistics partner, you will need to have a clear hypothesis, as its character plays a role in shaping what statistical tests you use. Hypotheses might be worded along the lines of: (a) The (intervention) will have a positive effect on intelligibility in (population); (b) The (intervention) will make a difference to intelligibility in (population); (c) The (intervention) will not have any effect on intelligibility in (population). These respectively are a directional, a non-directional and a null hypothesis.

In a *directional* or *one-tailed* hypothesis you are hypothesising that the change will be in a particular direction, for example that you expect the intervention will make things better. Alternatively, you may have no idea what the outcome will be and the intervention could have a positive or a negative outcome. This would be a *non-directional* or *two-tailed* hypothesis. The so-called null hypothesis is used when it is expected that there will be no change associated with the intervention.

What methods will I need to answer my question?

So far, we have talked about coming up with a clear, relevant question that is answerable within the scope of your resources and the data (potentially) available to you. However, there are many different ways of going about answering a question. Research design and methodology in evidence gathering is a huge topic and it is possible you might need guidance from both your NHS or university research design service and a statistician. This section introduces some common designs that might be suitable for answering clinical queries.

The common broader questions SLTs are likely to ask under the umbrella of this chapter title are: does my client's impairment improve after therapy? Or does this new intervention compare more favourably than another in making my client's impairment better? Managers might want to ask, 'Are our clients (from a specific caseload) improving at the impairment level?' Or, 'Do children who are seen for intervention in school improve more than when they are seen in clinic?'

As already discussed in Chapter 1, there are a variety of methods available to address this type of question, ranging from single case experimental designs through to RCTs across many centres. Each method has its strengths and weaknesses, depending on the nature of the question you are trying to answer. In an everyday clinical setting, the types of approaches you are most likely to be able to take to answer these questions are single case experimental designs, a case series design or perhaps a small group design. You may also wish to set up a way of collecting data from your caseload or client group, so you can look at the impact of your intervention at a future date or retrospectively. This would be particularly helpful if you wish to conduct an evaluation across the service or a part of it.

We have laid out below some guidelines in setting up a single case study, a case series design and a small group study. We then briefly address retrospective data collection which is expanded on in Chapter 8.

Single case studies

Single case experimental design (SCED) studies have been widely used in SLT and also constitute a large proportion (around 40%) of studies on brain impairment and published research on aphasia (Tate, McDonald, Perdices, Togther, Schulz, & Savage, 2008). RCTs, while being regarded as the gold standard, can present challenges; for example, powerful studies usually require a large number of participants. They also average out effects and so do not look at individual differences (see Thompson (2006) in the Further Reading section for a discussion on single subject designs). SCED studies are useful for preliminary investigations of new interventions. For example, you might read about a small study which shows some limited evidence for a particular approach to treating acquired apraxia of speech and, persuaded by the evidence, might like to evaluate with a new patient. SCEDs are also useful when studying rare conditions, where large numbers of participants are not feasible or for the early stages in testing out a new type of intervention. Tate et al. (2008) developed a SCED scale, a tool for appraising a single case experimental design study. Such appraisal tools are helpful to see what key factors are important when designing a robust SCED.

In a SCED, the participant acts as their own *control*; that is, there is usually a period where they do not receive intervention and where several measures are taken to establish a baseline/normal behaviour – this is the *control* phase. This helps us to see how behaviour changes when we introduce the IV or intervention – this is the *experimental* phase. We compare the measures from the two periods.

The evidence is more convincing if the behaviour drops back to the level it was prior to the experimental phase when the IV is withdrawn. This poses a problem with SLT intervention, in that we hope it has a lasting effect and therefore would not want to see a drop back to the baseline levels. A way round this might be to measure something else at the same time, that is similar to the DV, but which you do not expect your intervention to impact upon. For example, if you deliver rate control therapy and are sure, from your theoretical background, that this would not influence loudness levels in someone who has dysarthria, you could use loudness as a control by measuring this alongside rate control. Should you see stable scores in loudness throughout the phases, and changes in rate control during and following the experimental phase, then you can draw more convincing conclusions that your intervention impacted upon speaking rate.

Please see the Further Reading section for articles and books that go into further detail and will guide you in conducting a SCED. Single case studies, while perfect for determining whether treatment influences outcomes in individual clients, are always open to the criticism that they may not work for the next person or in another clinic with a different therapist. Moreover, they provide a low level of evidence and need to be supplemented by further studies. For this reason, alone or with other colleagues, you might wish to assemble a *case series* to determine whether this is the case or not.

Case series design

A case series design usually makes use of a small number of participants, where a SCED is applied to each individual. There is no separate control group and all participants receive the same assessments and intervention. In addition to individual outcomes, inferences are drawn from the collective data where trends across the group are identified. Case series designs are often used in pilot or feasibility studies and act as a base for developing higher level research. However, they can also be used to gather data across a service or client group. All that is required is the resolve and discipline to collect data in a systematic, controlled fashion and to assure that the intervention is administered in an identical manner across clients (and clinicians). This requires the intervention to be manualized; see the section on 'Getting to the detail' (p. 80) for more information. It is then possible to examine the series data to see how far the degree and patterns of change are replicated across individuals.

Small group design

In a small group design, as with an RCT, there are essentially two models of how you might organize comparisons between groups. You may have an independent group design or a matched group design. Within the matched group design you can have either two different sets of people who are matched one to one with each other, or you test/treat the same set of people under different conditions (this is also termed a repeated measures or crossover design).

The features you select for matching people across groups depend on your question and what factors you feel might exercise an influence on your treatment or test. The essential element though in a matched group design is that person 1 in group 1 will have an identical profile concerning all the key factors to person 1 in group 2; person 2 in group 1 will match person 2 in group 2 and so forth. It is clear from this that you will always end up with equal numbers in both groups.

In the repeated measures (so-called as you repeat the measures on the same people) version you don't have a problem with matching as you are using the same sample of participants for both measures. The disadvantage is that if you are testing exactly the same people under different conditions (e.g. with a semantic cue versus a phonemic cue) or have two treatment methods to compare, there is obviously going to be a potential learning or contamination effect that can distort your findings. A typical solution here (there are several other solutions if you wish to read up in the Further Reading section), is that you might have half of your participants receive condition 1 first followed by condition 2 whilst the other half receive condition 2 first and then condition 1.

In an independent group design, you have two different sets of people whom you have matched overall (e.g. mean age, ratio of girls to boys, average score on phonological awareness test), but other than that there is no necessity to have any one individual in group 1 being a carbon copy of someone in group 2. You can even have different numbers of people in the two groups.

Your statistics colleague will ask you whether you have an independent/unmatched or matched/repeated measures design, as the answer holds important implications for what statistical tests are used to analyze results.

Retrospective data collection

The answer to your question might already be sitting in your drawer. Are children more fluent after your treatment, now that you have introduced a particular type of intervention in your service? Is voice treatment outcome less favourable in smokers compared with non-smokers? You might work towards the answer by conducting a *retrospective* examination of the case notes of the last 50 patients or those within a certain time frame. A prerequisite to this, of course, is that the data have been recorded systematically in all notes, that the same assessments were applied to all participants in the same manner, and that the intervention was identical.

Using this method of evaluating intervention underlines the importance of discussion and decision-making amongst your team. A core set of data can be agreed upon and gathered for all service-users who are receiving a particular intervention. The assessments do not have to be limited to those outlined in the protocol, but a minimum set of data needs to be identified as necessary for the evaluation. See Chapter 8 for more detail on setting up this type of data collection.

Getting into the detail

You now need to make decisions about how you will set up your data collection, using the methods you have chosen or have been advised to use. This is really the start of developing your *protocol* where you document everything you are going to do and how you will do it in detail, so that you or anyone else can pick it up at any time and carry on.

Each decision needs to be thought out carefully and justified. The rationale for and methods of your intervention should be underpinned by your theoretical background. For instance, it should support your use of a given assessment task, your choice of intervention to modify the behaviour you are targeting and whether or not you can expect transfer and generalization. As is pointed out in Chapter 3, there may come a time when you find it difficult to remember the rationale behind a decision, so it is important to keep a record for reference.

A common criticism of articles on intervention is that the intervention is not sufficiently described. This makes it difficult for others to replicate it and means the data are difficult to evaluate and interpret, since one cannot conclude which elements of intervention may or may not be responsible for change. This underscores the importance of manualization of the assessment and therapy procedures. This ensures there is consistency in how the assessments and intervention are administered across clients and by different therapists. It also makes it possible to speculate on what components of the intervention might or might not be active in bringing about change. The following sections take a more detailed look at some of these issues.

Participants – which clients?

Think carefully about who is going to take part and from whom you are going to gather data. It is important for people reading about your research to set your results in context and understand, if the intervention works, for whom it is suitable or, if it isn't, why this might be so. You will need to develop *inclusion and exclusion criteria* so you are clear about whom you can invite into your study. Consider what factors about your clients might influence the outcome of your impairment intervention and blur its effects. We can probably divide factors into characteristics of the client that might determine whether to include them or not and logistical problems around study conduct.

Personal factors

When determining your inclusion and exclusion criteria, aspects to be considered could be, for example, age, gender, medical diagnosis, impairment severity and co-occurring diagnoses or comorbidities (such as memory problems, hearing loss, respiratory disease). There might also be other criteria, more specific to your particular client group, which relate to factors such as dental status, attention, fatigue, rapidly changing health status, time since last period of impairment therapy, and so on.

Be careful of using inclusion or exclusion criteria that are too stringent or searching for people with disorders that are very rare. For example, if you are looking for people who have apraxia of speech, the local pool could be quite extensive; but if you want to include only those who are six months post-stroke, who don't have an accompanying aphasia and who are over 70 years old, extensive will readily shrink to scarce. Participants bring with them idiosyncrasies, so they will vary. To make sure such variation does not contaminate any planned group comparisons, we typically randomize participants to receive the different intervention regimes. In theory, this distributes potential variability equally across the groups (or group halves if using a single group with a cross-over design). The bottom line and key rationale is to make different groups as comparable as possible on variables considered important. By doing this we know that our results reflect the effect of the IV and not just the natural difference that occurs between the two groups.

Even though your groups might be balanced at the start, some participants from one group might drop out before the completion of testing. This is referred to as attrition. The groups are therefore no longer directly comparable, so the results could be due to the resulting unequal group composition rather than the experimental variables. At the very minimum, in writing up, you must describe and account for 'drop outs'. Look carefully for possible reasons why this happened. They may relate to the demands you were placing on participants, for example, timing or location of appointments, or having to undergo several hours of tiring testing. It might relate to their attitude, for example, if they knew they were in the control group and so saw no point in turning up. At worst, you may need to redesign your study but at the least, you need to weigh up seriously the possible effects missing data have on your results and whether you can draw firm conclusions from them. A feasibility study is usually an early part of study set-up to 'eke' out these issues prior to commencing a large data collection.

Logistical factors

Logistical factors might prevent people from taking part in your study. These could include their availability (holidays, hospital appointments, co-ordination with your work days), transportation, health status, work and family commitments, etc. How can you overcome these? For example, someone may not be able to attend your clinic for an assessment, but you could visit them at home; it might be easier to assess some children at school. However, you will need to consider carefully if possible remedies will invalidate or contaminate the data you gather, for example, if you need a carefully controlled auditory environment.

Some factors can be difficult to control, for example, medication effects can influence performance in people who have Parkinson's disease. Since it would be unethical to ask participants to be non-medicated during a study, you need to consider methods for controlling for this to overcome or limit any influence on outcomes.

Baseline and outcome measures

Your primary outcome measure is the single most important measure that answers your central question. If the assessment doesn't actually measure the behaviour you want it to, and is not sufficiently sensitive to gauge the gradations of change you wish to capture, then it will undermine your whole project. Furthermore, application of assessments without attention to variables that could affect measurements will also render results dubious. It is therefore crucial that your primary outcome measure is valid and reliable and is applied at the correct junctures in a consistent fashion.

What and how shall I measure?

To answer this question, let's take an example: you might feel a measure of speaking rate (SR) will capture change in relation to your intervention and aims. First, you need to have a firm and transparent rationale for why this is the best variable to measure. Secondly, you need to decide how you are going to measure SR, as there are all sorts of ways to do this; for example, a rating scale, in syllables or words per minute, with or without pauses (what will constitute a pause?). You will also need to decide how you will deal with false starts and repetitions and what sort of speech sample you want to measure (reading or spontaneous speech?). You will also have to think about how you can obtain recordings of an appropriate quality and what might influence these (equipment, mouth to microphone distance, background noise, etc.).

How do I know my measures are valid and reliable?

The issue of *validity* centres around whether the chosen assessments are true measures of the variables selected for measurement. If they are not, then the answer you derive from your research will be invalid. Assessments include checklists, rating scales, clinicians' perceptual impressions, and similar, not just instrumental tools. For example, if a questionnaire purports to measure distress arising from a speech disorder, it should not confound that with distress arising from the underlying illness; if an assessment claims to measure motor speech performance, then the assessment items should represent speech production and not oral motor control.

The *reliability* of an assessment is the extent to which results are consistent if the assessment is repeated over time (test re-test reliability), with different raters (inter-rater reliability), or the same person rescoring the same data on a separate occasion (intra-rater reliability). To avoid learning effects and similar there are also sometimes matched versions of a test to use for reassessment. Reliability therefore also applies to whether the different versions of the test deliver acceptably equivalent measures (*internal consistency*).

Reliability is determined statistically, looking at the percentage agreement and relationship of scores. If you have a self-devised test, with no reliability data to hand, you might need to conduct your own inter- and intra-rater reliability checks. Test manuals should include a section on validity and reliability where you can find this information; be suspicious of tests that fail to supply this. Sometimes an outcome measure has not been published, but has become an accepted way of examining a particular variable. If this is the case, you will usually find evidence of its reliability in previous peer-reviewed papers where you will also find reviews of published assessments.

It's worth pointing out, though, that poor reliability does not preclude use of a measure if no other suitable metric is available. However, it does have serious implications when interpreting the results. Essentially, unless the size of change in your outcome test scores falls comfortably beyond the *margin of error*, one cannot confidently ascribe changes to the intervention or IV. Put simply, the margin of error is the difference in scores on a test you would get if you repeated it under the same conditions; that is, with the same participants, judges, same time of day, etc. See confidence intervals below for more detail on this issue.

Reliability can also be influenced by the number of items in a test; for example, transcription of single words could be a valid method to assess intelligibility. However, if only 5–10 items, or even 15–20 items are used, you might not be confident you have obtained a reliable picture of someone's capability or detected fine gradations of change. Scores that are converted into a percentage can make small changes look like big ones. For example, a step from 3/5 to 4/5 looks like a giant 20% leap forwards and a misplaced testament to successful therapy.

How many measures do I need?

Ideally, the burden of assessment on participants should be as light as possible. This chapter focuses on impairment outcomes but, as was raised in our introduction, you need to consider if an impairment measure truly reflects the clinical changes that are relevant. It may be appropriate to assess more broadly within an ICF perspective, looking additionally at activity and participation, to provide a more clinically relevant context.

Typically, you would have a measure of the primary outcome, the target of the intervention, but also measures of control variables to help you weigh up how far change is due to the intervention compared with a more general therapy effect; this was discussed in our section on SCEDs. You might also want to know whether the effects are item specific or if there has been generalization to different situations. Measures of other variables might also give you a broader picture. For example, in investigating the therapy effects targeted at voice quality in children with cerebral palsy, your primary outcome might be voice perturbation measures, but it could also be interesting to know whether changes in acoustic variables have an influence on perceptual variables, as measured through listener judgement and rating.

When do I need to conduct my assessments?

The number and timing of your assessments will depend upon your research design. If the degree of natural variation (for example, based on day-to-day, rapid developmental change, spontaneous recovery after stroke) is high, you need to achieve results in your post-intervention measure which go beyond this natural fluctuation in order to make claims that it is the intervention that has been responsible for change. If conducting a single case study, or case series, you will want to establish a good idea of how the behaviour fluctuates before you administer your intervention. Therefore, as well as the usual pre- and post-intervention measures, you would capture the picture of fluctuation by adopting a multiple baseline approach, that is, repeat your measures several times before introducing the intervention to get a picture of natural fluctuations in performance.

It is usually appropriate to see if the effects of intervention are maintained beyond treatment. For this reason, you should not only plan to conduct measures at termination of treatment but also at post-intervention stages over succeeding months.

Intervention – what intervention?

In this chapter we are addressing intervention that aims to change your client's *impairment,* so you need to think very carefully that your intervention focuses at the impairment level. Intervention in this sense might therefore be exercises, therapy tasks or advice on use of strategies.

Content of the intervention

Unless you can describe your intervention exactly, you cannot show that it has integrity and supports your evidence. Think through your intervention carefully and be clear about your rationale, which should be underpinned by an existing evidence base and your theoretical framework gleaned from your literature review. When delivering an intervention as part of a research investigation, make sure you keep a record of the intervention undertaken. This is because you may want to alter therapy tasks slightly during your intervention, such as increasing the complexity of the tasks if the client is improving or decreasing the speed of presentation of stimuli.

Delivery of the intervention

It is really important that the intervention is deliverable in a consistent manner;

for example, in each session, by each therapist, for each participant; and that it can be replicated. Consider whether you will need to use more than one therapist and how you will ensure that there is consistency amongst them when they provide intervention. The best thing is to write a manual of therapy ('manualize' in the current jargon).

Location of intervention

The location of the intervention may well be your independent variable, for example, home versus clinic. However, on a more practical level you need to make sure you have access to the accommodation you need. This is becoming increasingly important, as clinical space is now more commonly shared amongst colleagues and sometimes across disciplines. Make sure the room is sufficiently large enough if you are testing out group intervention and that it can accommodate wheelchairs or has any other facilities you may need.

If you are taking or listening to sound recordings as part of your assessments or therapy, make sure that the environment is quiet and, if possible, that the conditions are the same each time. If you are going to deliver intervention or assessments at home you need to be aware of potential disruptions such as callers, telephones, dogs barking, no table to sit at, etc. There may also be cost implications if you are likely to be doing more home visits or if a participant is expected to attend the clinic more often for a period of time. Make sure they can get to the clinic easily.

Some familiar biases in research

The factors described above are not the sole ones to be aware of in setting up your study. Biases can creep into the design, conduct, analysis and interpretation of your study at all stages.

The Hawthorn effect is a well-recognized source of bias in conducting research. This is the recognition that people may change their behaviour simply by having attention paid to them. Common solutions include comparing your intervention with a placebo condition (an intervention that should not influence the variables you wish to change) or a set of control measures, as outlined above, that you predict should remain uninfluenced by your intervention.

The Pygmalion effect, or self-fulfilling prophesies, might also influence your outcomes. This involves the power of expectation on behalf of the participant or the researcher. For example, if the researcher expects a person to do poorly (without even telling them), lo and behold they do poorly. Common solutions to this conundrum entail careful consideration and standardisation of information about interventions and careful wording of instructions. Ideally, one should have an independent colleague carry out baseline and outcome measures, blind to which intervention an individual has received. Therapists should, ideally, also be blind to expectations about an intervention. This may be easy when the intervention is a drug, but is clearly impractical where active behavioural interventions are concerned. Where resources permit, a solution is to randomize therapists to deliver the different interventions as well as to randomize participants in receiving them. The bottom line is that the researcher should be aware of the influence of expectations and take all possible practical steps to avoid it.

Experimenter bias lurks in many corners. There may be something about the experimenter or the way they conduct the experiment that influences the outcome. This could be their gender, age, language or body language, the way they speak or the atmosphere they create.

Situational or instrumental effects can undermine comparisons and conclusions. Participants can be well matched, but if they are tested under differing conditions this could influence the 'fairness' of the comparison. For example, you may conduct an assessment in quiet conditions for one participant and in rather distracting conditions for another. Or you might make top-class sound recordings to assess intelligibility, but then undermine it all by playing them back to listeners through poor quality headphones.

Two common biases in testing are fatigue and learning effects. In the former, participants can perform more poorly on later items as they lose attention or tire; in the latter, participants may perform better later on in the assessment, or on retesting, as they gain insight into what is required. Typical solutions would be to randomize the order in which subtests are conducted within a test. Alternatively, you can simply have half the participants following the order item one to 50, the others starting at 50 and going back to one. The same could apply when it comes to people scoring your tests.

Textbooks on research design will detail the solutions to these biases, how to avoid them in the first place or how to control for them if they are unavoidable. See the Further Reading section for more information.

Preparing for the unexpected

It would be nice if data collection and research studies always ran smoothly but, sadly, this is hardly ever the case. Even when careful thought has been given to all aspects of the data collection and the design, unexpected issues arise. It is always a good idea to try as best you can to imagine what could happen when 'real life' intervenes. For example, if you have decided to administer x number of sessions over x number of days or weeks, but your client or clients become ill – or indeed you do? What if your patient bursts into tears half way through your assessment? You will need to think how flexible you can be with your assessments and intervention whilst still remaining true to your protocol. The 'what if?' question is a useful one to ask yourself before, and throughout, developing your protocol. This will help you prepare for potential set-backs, have plans for how to resolve them as much as possible and allow you to still have helpful results to show at the end.

Ethical issues

Sometimes when you are developing methods for gathering data, questions arise that challenge an ethical issue. In terms of evaluating the effects of intervention on impairment, there are several that you may come across. For example, fluctuating performance could be associated with unstable medication effects, but there are ethical issues of withdrawing or delaying this to obtain stability in our measures. Others we may encounter are delaying intervention, such that we can take multiple baselines or offering a *placebo* therapy before actual therapy commences.

Sometimes there is no evidence that, for example, delaying treatment will be detrimental, in which case we could argue reasonably that delay will bring no harm. Sometimes ethical issues relate to our proposed methods, for example, is it ethical to demand a videofluoroscopy examination of someone who does not actually need it, or to carry out lengthy tiring assessment batteries with someone soon after stroke, or withdraw a child from class for your assessments/treatment?

If you are truly conducting research, as opposed to audit or service evaluation, then you must take your protocol through an ethics committee. If you are gathering evidence on service delivery, then you still need to be ethically mindful. As has been pointed out in Chapter 2, involving client focus groups to assist you in developing your protocol, information sheets and consent forms is not only a requirement for research, but a huge help.

Analysis of data

Before moving on to this brief overview of data analysis, we stress that you must consider how you are going to analyze your results *before* you start your project. This is to ensure your methods will allow you to answer your question and that you are collecting the right type of data in a manner to permit you to arrive at a valid and reliable answer. There is nothing worse than having collected a set of data that you cannot then analyze after all your hard work. There are two broad avenues to data processing: descriptive statistics and inferential statistics.

Descriptive statistics

Descriptive statistics describe what the data look like. They can provide a measure of *central tendency* (the 'average') such as the *mean* (arithmetic average), the *mode* (most frequent value) and the *median* (the middle value). Measures of central tendency are meaningless, though, without an indication of the spread of the data. Your choice of the type of spread you report will depend on the kind of data you have generated and whether or not it is normally distributed. To describe the spread of values, you can use the *range* of the data values, the *interquartile range* (IQR) which is the range of data held in the middle 50% of the values, and/or the *standard deviation*.

Inferential statistics

Our descriptive statistics might look pretty convincing, but to obtain more substantial evidence of the outcome of our work we need, if we can, to use inferential analyses. If our study design is appropriate and procedures have been carried out correctly, these will show us if any difference is statistically significant – that is, not just due to chance.

The international convention recognized to be the cut-off point between chance and statistical significance is equal to or less than 1 in 20, that is, 5%. This is expressed as p (for *probability*), so, for example, 5% probability would be expressed as $p = 0.05$. You can apply stricter criteria looking for differences that have a probability of occurring less than 1% ($p = <0.01$). The closer p moves to 0 the greater the statistical significance; the closer to 1, the less there is any change beyond chance.

The p value is not so much an absolute value as an approximation of the probability. It is therefore more informative to include also an indication of the margin of error there might be in this estimation. This is called the *confidence interval* (CI). You therefore might report, for example, mean = 62.7 (CI 59.8–64.6). Here we can see that the estimated value of the mean is 62.7 but we know that really it could be anywhere between 59.8 and 64.6. The greater the interval, the less certain one is of the true value. For further information on these and other statistical terms, good starter references are Hinton (2004) and Miller (2006); see Further Reading.

Summary

Within a clinical context it is possible to see if your intervention impacts upon your client's impairment. With careful planning, you can do this with a single client, several clients or a whole caseload. The crucial first step is to really understand what it is you want to know and refine that broader clinical query into a manageable question. Your literature review will help you rationalize your choice of intervention and outcome measures and help you to see how others have tried to overcome some of the obstacles you may face. Careful consideration should be given to ensure you choose an appropriate, valid and reliable assessment for your primary outcome measure. To ensure the intervention is carried out consistently across clients and therapists, it is best to manualize the intervention. It is important to seek the support of others who can help you, particularly with your design and analysis. While developing your protocol, you should be aware of any ethical issues that arise, whether conducting a research project or a service evaluation, and always understand the limitations of your findings.

References

Hartelius, L. & Miller, N. (2010) The ICF framework and its relevance to the assessment of people with motor speech disorders. In A. Lowit and R. Kent (Eds) *Assessment of Motor Speech Disorders*. San Diego: Plural, pp. 1–20.

Tate, R. L., McDonald, S., Perdices, M., Togther, L., Schulz, R., & Savage, S. (2008) Rating the methodological quality of single-subject designs and *n*-of-1 trials: Introducing the single-case experimental design (SCED) scale. *Neuropsychological Rehabilitation* **18:4**, 385–401.

World Health Organisation (2007) *International Classification of Functioning, Disability and Health*. http://www.who.int/classifications/icf/

Further reading

Single case design

Barlow, D., Nock, M., & Hersen, M. (2009) *Single Case Experimental designs: Strategies for Studying Behavior for Change* (3rd edition). Boston: Pearson Education Inc.

Beeson, P. M. & Robey, R. R. (2006) Evaluating single-subject treatment research: Lessons learned from the aphasia literature. *Neuropsychology Review* **16:4**, 161–169.

Thompson, C. K. (2006) Single subject controlled experiments in aphasia: The science and the state of the science. *Journal of Communication Disorders* **39:4**, 266–291.

General research

Dollaghan, C. (2004) Evidence-based practice in communication disorders: What do we know, and when do we know it? *Journal of Communication Disorders* **37:5**, 391–400.

Dollaghan, C. A. (2007) *The Handbook for Evidence-based Practice in Communication Disorders*. Baltimore: Brookes Publishing Co.

Elmes, D., Kantowitz, B. H., & Roediger, III. H. L. (2011) *Research Methods in Psychology* (9th edition). Belmont: Wadsworth.

Finn, P., Bothe, A. K., & Bramlett, R. E. (2005) Science and pseudoscience in communication disorders: Criteria and applications. *American Journal of Speech-Language Pathology* **14:Aug**, 172–186.

Hamilton, J. (2005) The answerable question and a hierarchy of evidence. *Journal of the American Academy of Child and Adolescent Psychiatry* **44:6**, 596–600.

Horner, S., Rew, L., & Torres, R. (2006) Enhancing intervention fidelity: A means of strengthening study impact. *Journal for Specialists in Paediatric Nursing* **11:2**, 80–89.

Hicks, C. M. (2009) *Research Methods for Clinical Therapists: Applied Project Design and Analysis* (5th edition). Oxford: Churchill Livingston, Elsevier Ltd.

Moncher, F. J. & Prinz, R. J. (1991) Treatment fidelity in outcome measures. *Clinical Psychology Review* **11:3**, 24–266.

Moule, P. & Hek, G. (2011) *Making Sense of Research: An Introduction for Health and Social Care Practitioners* (4th edition). London: Sage Publications.

Neale, J. (Ed) (2009) *Research Methods for Health and Social Care*. Basingstoke: Palgrave Macmillan.

Robson, C. (2006) *How to Do a Research Project: A Guide for Undergraduate Students*. London: Blackwell.

Wambaugh, J. & Bain, B. (2002) Making your research an integral part of your clinical practice. *ASHA Leader*, November 19.

Measurement and statistics

Gravetter, F. J. & Wallnau, L. B. (2008) *Essentials of Statistics for the Behavioural Sciences* (6th edition). Belmont: Thomson/Wadsworth.

Hinton, P. (2004) *Statistics Explained* (2nd edition). Hove: Routledge.

Miller, S. (2009) *Experimental Design and Statistics* (2nd edition). London: Routledge, Taylor Francis Group.

Streiner, D. L. & Norman, G. R. (2008) *Health Measurement Scales: A Guide to their Development and Use* (4th edition). Oxford: Oxford University Press.

Turkstra, L. S., Coelho, C., & Ylvisaker, M. (2005) The use of standardized tests for individuals with cognitive-communication disorders. *Seminars in Speech and Language* **26:4** 215–221.

Resources

American Speech and Hearing Association: excellent summary of evidence-based medicine techniques – see in particular the sections on formulating questions, developing methodologies, evaluating evidence. There is a great web-based tutorial. http://www.asha.org/research/

Cochrane Collaboration: This provides authoritative reviews on all aspects of health care (not just communication disorders). This website will give you an impression of the sheer breadth of this collaboration and also introduce you to how systematic reviews work and what kind of evidence is taken as proof, or not, of efficacy. http://www.cochrane.org/cochrane-reviews

Levels of evidence

In the different books, articles and guidelines you read, you will see reference to the notion of 'levels of evidence'. This refers to the strength of the evidence provided by a particular study in relation to a clinical question. Generally, strength ranges from expert opinion (not backed up by facts and figures) through to hard facts and figures based on large-scale trials comparing different forms of treatment/delivery, or studies that have combined the results of many trials into meta-analyses. The problem is that not everyone employs the same rating scales for indicating strength of evidence; the websites listed below detail the more widely-employed scales.

http://www.cebm.net/index.aspx?o=1025

http://www.patient.co.uk/doctor/Different-Levels-of-Evidence-(Critical-Reading).htm

http://www.essentialevidenceplus.com/product/ebm_loe.cfm?show=oxford

Appendix

Answers to DV and IV questions:

1. DV vocabulary skills; IV location of 8-year-olds.

2. DV degree of stuttering; IV the language used.

3. DV amount of eye contact; IV whether or not intervention had taken place.

5 How does my intervention affect my client's quality of life?

Chris Markham

Learning outcomes

By the end of this chapter, you will be able to:

- Recognize the value of quality of life (QoL) as a health outcome measure
- Define and understand the competing definitions of QoL
- Recognize the variety of methods available when researching QoL
- Discuss the validity of the range of QoL measurement methods
- Design a QoL study

Introduction

This chapter discusses gathering evidence on the impact of communication needs and speech and language therapy intervention on a client's Quality of Life (QoL). It begins by showing how QoL assessment can contribute to client care and introduces definitions of QoL. The chapter then goes on to look at some of the key issues around QoL as an outcome measure and to discuss some of the approaches a busy clinician might consider when searching for and generating QoL evidence. The final sections of the chapter focus on central issues to be considered when designing a project to develop QoL evidence for people with speech, language and communication needs.

QoL is something talked about on a daily basis, across all societies and cultures and, interestingly, is an idea that has been around for over 2000 years, when ancient Greek philosophers tried to decide what it was. Despite different individuals and societies accepting that there is this thing called QoL, we still don't have one complete understanding of what it is. This is because QoL means different things, to different people, at different times (Fayers & Machin, 2007). For example, QoL can be used to refer to a nation's wealth, the built environment and an individual's satisfaction with their life, ideas of which change over time and place. As this chapter will show, because of these different ideas about QoL, but a shared perception of the ideal, it is challenging to both define and then measure it, but attempts to do so within health and social care can provide important outcomes to clients, clinicians, commissioners and policymakers alike.

It is now widely acknowledged that the personal burden of health conditions cannot be fully described by impairment-based measures such as the degree of language delay, physical and/or cognitive abilities. Psychosocial factors and the individual's perception of their health status and its impact on their daily lives are increasingly seen as important in a person's healthcare. In fact, the World Health Organisation's (WHO) International Classification of Functioning, Disability and Health (ICF) now encourages the evaluation and support of all areas of service users' lives (World Health Organisation, 2002). QoL assessment can be seen as an example of how the WHO's aspiration is being met globally, particularly their principles of *Activity* and *Participation*.

QoL assessment therefore has the potential to target and capture broader therapeutic aims and outcomes in a systematic and client-centred way. It provides a holistic understanding of an individual's condition and therefore a greater number of alternatives to managing it (Bowling, 2001). Indeed, some authors maintain that assessment of QoL variables is essential within the provision and evaluation of complex interventions such as speech and language therapy, where it also provides a formal method for the assessment and inclusion of the client's perspective in their care (Fayers & Machin, 2007).

QoL assessment enables clinicians to set patient-centred goals and, in some cases, could be more likely to bring about and demonstrate clinical effectiveness. For example, for those clients who have plateaued in their speech and language therapy or who have a more negative prognosis for their communication skills, QoL assessment provides an opportunity to address more holistic aspects of communication needs that affect clients' life experience. Indeed, for some clients, improvements in emotional and social functioning are as important as changes in their physical or cognitive status (Eiser & Morse, 2001). Moreover, in the case of speech and language therapy, clients with chronic communication difficulties have a higher incidence of psychosocial and emotional problems that impact on their condition and QoL.

In the case of a complex intervention such as speech and language therapy, where treatment effects may be small, QoL data can be a relevant and persuasive outcome to clients and commissioners alike. Similarly, there is a body of evidence that demonstrates the impact on QoL for the carers of people with communication or related needs. For example, research has shown that parents of children with developmental needs and carers of adults with communication needs can all experience negative QoL as a consequence of their caring responsibilities. Speech and language interventions that target carers, then, can equally be evaluated for the benefits they could have for carers themselves.

What are the clinical issues or challenges?

Although our professional guidelines encourage the inclusion of QoL assessment, there are numerous challenges and few methods to do this. One of the first challenges is finding a workable definition of QoL.

Definitions of QoL

Despite the rise in the use of QoL in both healthcare and the wider world, it remains a universally undefined concept (Eiser & Morse, 2001). Happiness, life satisfaction, wellbeing, self-actualisation and fulfilment are just a few of the terms that are currently used by academics, politicians and professionals to discuss QoL. This has led some researchers in the field to conclude that the number of definitions in existence are now so numerous and varied that there is no hope of reaching a single, comprehensive overview of what QoL is and consequently no standard method to measure it. Although we all like the idea of QoL, quotes such as the following remind us of the importance of defining it first:

> The term 'quality of life' is great in speeches, but when it is given the stature of a research concept, it becomes an uncertain tool, unless it is controlled by a precise definition and rigorous discipline in thought and word (Wolfensberger, 1994, p. 318).

When considering what QoL is, a useful starting point is the World Health Organisation, that defines health as 'a state of complete physical, mental and social well-being and not merely the absence of disease' (World Health Organisation, 1947). The WHO therefore defines QoL as an individual's perception of their position in life in the context of the culture and value systems in which they live and in relation to their goals, expectations, standards and concerns (World Health Organisation QoL Group, 1993). This definition suggests that QoL is affected in complex ways – by a person's physical health, psychological state, level of independence and social relationships – and is a useful guide when considering the impact of communication needs on a person's life.

Similarly, research using 'concept analyses' which attempt to clarify abstract ideas such as QoL, has revealed the following features of a consistent definition of QoL:

- QoL is an evaluation of an individual's current life circumstances

- QoL is multidimensional

- QoL is value based and dynamic

- QoL comprises subjective and objective factors

- QoL is most reliably measured by the individual themselves, using subjective indicators

Considering the role of speech and language therapy, in addition to satisfaction with life, some authors have also added the dimensions *normal life, achievement of personal goals* and *happiness* to definitions of QoL. Normal life is defined as the absence of limitations in functional abilities such as daily communication with others and achievement of personal goals related to the discrepancy between an individual's goals in life and their ability to achieve them. These ideas therefore suggest that an individual's QoL is enhanced if they are personally fulfilled, because the gap between expectation and reality is small or even non-existent. Of course, communication needs impact directly on any individual's ability to achieve their life goals and therefore impact on their quality of life.

Quality of life and speech, language and communication needs

Looking at the discussion above, it is possible to see how speech, language and communication needs can be better understood and supported using knowledge of QoL. Research and practice utilizing QoL in speech and language therapy is in its infancy, but some valuable and interesting evidence exists. For example, research with communication-impaired adults showed that the QoL of people living with long-term aphasia was significantly affected by, amongst other things, emotional distress, reduced participation in activities, problems affecting family life, isolation and low self-confidence (Hilari, Byng,

Lamping, & Smith, 2003). Another study by Klugman and Ross (2002) found that a number of adults with multiple sclerosis not only experienced speech and language problems, but also that 62% of those with speech, language and communication needs (SLCNs) reported this as having a [negative] impact on their QoL.

Within the paediatric arena, Connor, Cohen, Theis, Thibeault, Heatley, and Bless (2008) demonstrated that voice disorders in childhood had a negative impact on children's social development and self-esteem as well as their communicative effectiveness. Emotional factors were prominent in the responses of school-aged children and young people in their study, who reported that their voice difficulties often limited their participation in important events and led to feelings of anger, sadness, and frustration. Within a more diverse population of children and young people with SLCNs and their carers, Markham, Van Laar, Gibbard, and Dean (2009) provide findings from an analysis of focus group interviews, where participants identified, amongst other things, *individual success*, *reduced frustration* and *participation at school* as priorities in improving their QoL.

Despite these examples, although we know a great deal about QoL generally, within speech and language therapy there is only an emerging literature, which makes it an ideal opportunity for clinicians wishing to generate evidence. The starting point for this could be discussions with service users, their families and other stakeholders about communication difficulties and their impact on QoL and how speech and language management can contribute to improving life experience. Alternatively, you might use an existing QoL measure and use it with a client to measure their life satisfaction. Either way, one of the most important points to bear in mind is the importance of defining and justifying the definition of QoL that is used.

In addition to a clear definition of QoL, one of the early and important steps in gathering evidence is a comprehensive literature review to see what has already been accomplished.

What do we already know about it?

Conducting a review of the literature is a critical step in generating useful evidence. A literature review could be used to identify what is already known about the life experiences and priorities of clients who have SLCNs, and also to explore the variety of methods used to generate QoL evidence. When searching the QoL literature, it is equally important to consider the diversity of QoL and the terms surrounding it. For example, in order to maximize the number of relevant articles you find, include terms such as *health related quality of life, quality of life, self-reported, subjective, wellbeing, life satisfaction* and *functional health*. There will also be others you will need to identify according to the client population you will be working with and the research method you will use. Also, think carefully about the client population you are interested in; it is a good idea to maximize your search potential by widening its scope using broad terms. For example, you might include both the specific term *aphasia* and the broader term *stroke*, or the specific term *language delay* and more generally *learning difficulty*. The idea is not to narrow the search using specific terms that might not reveal any evidence, but to open it up to all potentially relevant publications that will help you understand and plan your project.

Once you have identified relevant literature, it will be necessary to appraise both its quality and value to your area of interest. Chapter 3 provides detailed advice on how to conduct a literature review and appraise the evidence; however, here are some tips with reference to reviewing QoL studies:

- Is there a clear and justifiable definition of QoL guiding the research?

- Was the research qualitative, quantitative or a mixture of both?

- Is the research population defined, so you know whether the results can be applied to the population that interests you??

- If a QoL measure has been used for data collection, was it reliable and valid?

- Was there potential for bias? For example, who provided the data on QoL, the client or a proxy?

With answers to these questions, decisions can be made about the value of the studies identified to your area of interest. Finally, it is worth considering the authors' recommendations for future research – this could be your opportunity!

Refining the question

There are two key elements in developing a research or service evaluation question in this area: first, the population of interest and, second, the definition of QoL that you will use. With reference to the clients you are interested in, this could include numerous demographic characteristics, for example: gender, age and occupation, their speech and language diagnoses, other medical diagnoses and also the type of intervention they might be receiving from a speech and language therapy service. With reference to your definition of QoL, as we have seen above, this is challenging because it is both multifactorial and there are competing definitions and terms used in the field. The important point here is to develop an operational definition of what you mean by QoL and use it to drive your work. Your Patient and Public Involvement (PPI) group could be very helpful here.

What methods will I need to answer my question?

The methods you use to answer your question really depend on what question you are asking and what evidence is already out there. For example, there are already a few QoL measures that can be used with people who have communication disorders, which means you could plan a small descriptive study using one of these measures to profile the QoL of a client or group of clients you are working with. Alternatively, there is much still to learn about the specific QoL experiences that people with different communication needs have. With respect to this, there are good opportunities for clinicians to consider developing evidence based on focus group or interview data, exploring with clients and all types of carers, the QoL implications of their communication difficulty.

The numerous research methods can be distinguished according to whether they will involve qualitative or quantitative approaches, although more complicated evidence can be generated using both approaches in a mixed method study. If you are aiming for a rich, descriptive insight into a client's QoL, from their point of view, then a qualitative, minimally structured approach should be taken. This could range from an open discussion with a client regarding their life situation to the use of an interview guide developed from ideas within the literature about QoL. A quantitative approach might make use of a validated QoL questionnaire which will provide data that can be quantified and subjected to statistical analyses. This could be used to present evidence of QoL of whole client groups.

Evidence generated using standardized QoL measures could be used to compare an individual's QoL with their impairment-based assessment findings in a case study, or administered to a group of clients with the same diagnoses in a cross sectional descriptive study of their life satisfaction. Other possibilities include correlating the QoL of different client groups with themselves or nonimpaired populations or, more commonly comparing a client or clients' QoL before and after an episode of speech and language management.

This short section introduces you to ideas about the overall design of a QoL study and the clinical possibilities of QoL research, whereas the following section addresses, in detail, some of the key research methods that need to be considered within a study design.

Getting into the detail

Defining the population

One of the first practicalities for speech and language populations relates to common definitions of QoL, which place subjective perceptions at the heart of what QoL is. This could be a challenge, because it will require client reports of their perceived personal and social wellbeing. Therefore, in order to collect data, clients could be required to have, at the least, independent and coherent communication or literacy skills. These requirements, however, narrow the potential field of client populations you could work with; they would certainly preclude clients with severe cognitive, physical and linguistic difficulties, who are arguably the very people whose QoL you want to enhance. In this case, it is possible – and there are examples in the further reading – where creative and compensatory research methods can be used to profile the QoL of such groups. However, more innovative ways of accessing clients' views or using indirect measures of QoL are a compromise, which in particular raises the potential for bias in a study. This is because the validity of proxy reports of a person's QoL or functional skills or non-standardized assessments of it, is reduced and you will be less confident in the results you obtain. This should be borne in mind when you review the literature

Sampling

Once you have identified a target population, you will need to take a sample of it for your study. Sampling participants for a QoL study requires similar considerations to sampling in any other study. This is really a question of compromise, between generating valid evidence and what you can realistically achieve with the time and resources available. A qualitative approach will require that you think about important client characteristics using a purposive sampling strategy, whereas in a quantitative approach your aim will be to reduce potential bias from the many confounders involved in QoL measurement (Ritchie & Lewis, 2005; Fayers & Machin, 2007). If you intend to provide a profile of a client or client group's QoL, then it should be representative. This means it should be an accurate reflection of the person's or group's QoL, which minimizes the potential for bias. Although this can be achieved through random sampling, often of large groups, it is challenging to a busy clinician. In this case, clinicians might opt to choose other, more 'convenient' methods of sampling, which are more achievable, but have the potential for bias that should be considered when evaluating and presenting your results.

Data collection

How data will be collected relates to the question you are asking and whether you are using a quantitative or qualitative approach. QoL data can be collected wherever convenient to both the clinician and client and could include a clinic, school, workplace or a client's own home. Indeed, as with any measurement of health, it is advisable to consider where a client will feel most relaxed to consider and respond to questions about their QoL.

If you are going to adopt a qualitative approach, you should read Chapter 6 alongside this one, and remember to take an audio recording device and ensure there will be a power supply if you need one and no excessive sound interference. There are no particular restrictions to when data can be collected, although you should be sensitive to the fact that most QoL measures are cross-sectional and, as such, represent a snapshot of a person's QoL, so significant life events around the time of measurement may influence your findings.

Measuring QoL

This section looks at methods you can use to explore and describe the QoL of clients and groups of them using firstly quantitative and then qualitative methods. Bowling (2001) provides a useful introduction and summary of the key methods in QoL assessment, ranging from subjective interpretations of an individual's life quality to objective economic analyses of the quantity of life quality. Quality of life measures, arguably, lie somewhere between the two, depending on their use of subjective or objective question items.

Perhaps the most extreme methods of objective measurement are quality-adjusted life years (QALYs) and disability-adjusted life years (DALYs). You will certainly read about these in preparing any QoL research, but might not always use them yourself. QALYs and DALYs contribute to understanding healthcare needs and interventions by providing a standardized unit of measurement to calculate the ratio of cost between different treatments with respect to their varying levels of effectiveness. However, the usefulness of QALYs and DALYs is debated, because there is no evidence to show that the units of measurement used have any relationship to the judgements of individuals suffering from the conditions themselves (Bowling, 2001). They are just too objective.

A more suitable approach to objective clinical measurement would be to use a published QoL measure. Many of these standardized measures, used in both research and clinical care, are founded on the principle that no two people experience the same condition and treatment of it in identical ways. They should have been developed respecting this important maxim in QoL measurement and should also have information about their development and use. Standard QoL measures are typically questionnaires that are client or carer completed. Ideally, a client should provide their own responses, but in cases where a person has no independent communication, then carer-completed measures may be necessary.

Alternatively, you could use qualitative ways of assessing and/or understanding QoL. Qualitative approaches are less structured than standardized measures, but are equally valid. Again, Chapter 6 provides greater detail about qualitative research methods, but one-to-one interviews or focus groups with clients and or carers can be effectively used to explore clients' QoL. One of the most important resources will be a topic guide, developed from existing evidence in the literature, used to prompt and probe QoL experiences and generate highly internally valid evidence of those individuals' QoL. Of course, you could combine qualitative and quantitative approaches in a 'mixed method' study of QoL. Bowling (2001) discusses one example in a description of human judgement analysis. Human judgement analysis uses open-ended questions to encourage participants to list the most important areas of their lives in relation to their QoL. Participants in these studies are then required to rate their current status on the dimension identified using visual analogue scales.

To conclude this section, it will be useful to reflect back on your research aim when selecting a research method. For example, objective measures may be more suitable when convincing groups such as commissioners, colleagues and academics, whereas more subjective approaches to QoL evidence could provide client-centred data with greater value to clinical management and client and carer feedback.

How do I choose my measure?

If you choose a quantitative design, before selecting and administering a measure of QoL, it is important to understand how it has been developed and what it aims to measure. Health outcome scales, such as QoL measures, should be developed using rigorous methods, because important treatment or policy decisions might be based on the outcomes measured by them (Fayers & Machin, 2007). An excellent source of both measures and information about them can be found on the Patient-Reported Outcome and Quality of Life Instruments Database (PROQOLID) website, where you can search a database of QoL measures according to pathology and/or population and find information about their development (see Resources at the end of this chapter).

Understanding how measures have been created will help you decide which of the many QoL measures available you might use to generate some evidence from a clinical population. Initially, you might be concerned to choose measures that demonstrate the highest levels of scientific credibility, but another important consideration will be a the method of administration. Many measures are self-completed or require an individual to have the capacity to understand questions spoken to them and respond independently. For speech and language clinicians working with clients who may have literacy and expressive and receptive communication needs, this could preclude some forms of QoL measure, or at least require modification of them, which could invalidate findings. Again, you might like to review some of the work that can be found in the further reading at the end of this chapter, to see examples of client reported functional outcomes. In particular, recent works in the field of aphasia, such as Long, Hesketh, Paszek, Booth and Bowen (2008) and Hilari et al. (2003) could be of interest; also Roulstone and McLeod's (2011) recent book focusing on children and young people.

Creating a QoL measure

The initial stages in the development of a new measure involve identifying exactly what will be measured. This crucial stage should include the advice of experts, information from within the related literature and, importantly, the inclusion of service users. There are then two methods for designing a QoL measure; these are either the clinimetric or psychometric approaches. You don't need an exhaustive understanding of these two terms, but should look out for them when working and reading in this area. What is important is that the two approaches lead to measures with different levels of validity, which many authors feel are greater following psychometric approaches. This is because clinimetric designs rely on the intuitive judgements of patients and clinicians to select question items for inclusion in a new measure, whereas psychometric designs use statistical techniques to select question items according to their covariance with one another. Clinimetric designs are consequently criticised for their *ad hoc* methods of item selection that are less likely to generalize to the wider clinical population (Fayers & Machin, 2007).

Validity and reliability

Reliability and validity are important considerations in any research outcomes and high levels of both give users of research data more confidence in the findings. Reliability is the consistency and repeatability of a measure and consists of internal consistency, test-retest reliability and inter-observer reliability (Fayers & Machin, 2007). Internal consistency tells you whether each question is contributing significantly to overall QoL scores, whereas test-retest and inter-observer reliability inform you of a measure's consistency over time and between different raters respectively. These three reliabilities are particularly important to QoL measures and you should check for them in any measure you use.

Evidence of a measure's validity tells you how accurately it measures the definition of QoL underpinning it. Validity is the most fundamental and important characteristic of a measure, because inferences drawn from a valid test are appropriate, meaningful and useful. There are three areas of validity important to QoL measures: content, criterion and construct validities. Content validity is simply whether or not a measure actually measures all of the important components of QoL, discussed above. Tests of content validity establish the extent to which a measure represents the content of interest, in our case QoL. Criterion validity is a question of how well the measure you are interested in provides similar results to other similar (QoL) measures and, finally, estimates of construct validity indicate how well a measure scales QoL and nothing else. You do not want to use a measure that is inaccurate and, in addition to QoL, also captures other aspects of a person's health.

Generalizability of QoL measures

Quality of life scales are distinguished as either generic or disease-specific. Generic measures are overall scales of QoL, which have not been designed for use with populations experiencing a particular disease or condition and can therefore be used with different population groups. Consequently, the main advantage of generic measures is found in their wider generalizability. Moreover, interventions can affect outcomes that are not condition specific and generic measures could pick up QoL changes that were not anticipated and thus not included in disease-specific measures. On the other hand, disease-specific measures are developed with specific populations in mind and are not intended for general application, although they should be general enough to apply to different subpopulations with the same condition (Fayers & Machin, 2007). Their main advantage is increased validity and sensitivity, because they are more likely than generic measures to detect small, but clinically significant, changes in health status or severity of disease.

Who will measure?

In addition to deciding whether to use a generic or specific measure, there comes the crucial question of who should rate an individual's QoL. If we accept that QoL is a person's perception of their physical, social and psychological health, then it is the individual who should rate their QoL. However, there are some measures that are designed to be completed by another, such as a parent or clinician, with the justification that the final results are more objective. This is known as 'proxy' reporting and suffers from all of the inaccuracies occasionally heard by speech and language clinicians listening to third party descriptions of clients' communication skills. Proxy response is an important point, because it may be the only method available for some clients with SLCNs, typically those with the greatest SLCNs and possibly the lowest QoL. Yet research tells us that proxy reporting leads to biased findings that often bear no relationship to how the person actually feels, even when the proxy rater knows the respondent well.

This section has discussed some key considerations to make when choosing a QoL measure to answer a research question. Below is a summary of these if you decide to use an existing measure:

- Is there evidence of the measure's reliability and validity?

- Who responds to the measure, a client or proxy respondent?

- Is there the potential for confusing vocabulary or response categories? (Some response categories use Likert [level of agreement] scales of 5, 7 or more which some clients may find confusing and difficult to utilize.)

- Is there the potential for distressing questions or responses? (For example, those relating to success and relationships; prepare for what you will do if the client becomes distressed or whose score indicates poor QoL.)

- Is the time taken to complete the assessment a burden on the client? (For example, will a further appointment be necessary to complete the measure and, if so, will it invalidate the findings?)

- Is normative data provided and, if not, how will you use the results in a meaningful way?

The answers to these questions should be found in the technical manuals supplied with the QoL measure or in publications about how the measure has been designed. Understanding the measure and its design will help you in later stages of a project where you will manage, analyze and report your data.

Managing the data

The next stage is to decide how to manage and analyze the data you collect. There are some shared principles regarding the management of either qualitative or quantitative data. All data will need to be securely held, for example, in locked filing cabinets and within password-protected computers. Quantitative data management will include coding data and inputting it into one of the numerous analytical software packages available. Coding quantitative data is simply a process of assigning consistent numerical codes to participants' responses to whatever measure has been used, typically Likert scales. In this coded form, the data are then available for statistical analysis. Similarly, qualitative data, such as interview and focus group recordings, will need to be anonymized, transcribed verbatim and synthesized with any memos made during the interview in preparation for its analysis.

Analysis

Earlier, this chapter discussed quantitative and qualitative approaches to QoL research. Each methodology requires a different approach to analysis, which will also be guided by your original research question. For example, quantitative studies, where you may be profiling a single group's QoL or demonstrating that your intervention has improved QoL to a commissioning panel, may make use of descriptive statistics. Descriptive statistics allow you to illustrate QoL differences and changes in it using graphs, pie charts and percentages.

However, you might be more ambitious and wish, for example, to evaluate statistically significant variations in the QoL of different client groups or client groups compared with non-disordered populations. In these examples, you will need to use inferential statistics. These types of statistics allow you to analyze your data in more complex ways, but require much more data management and understanding of analysis, which Chapter 4 explores in more detail. If this seems daunting, you should consider contacting a statistician, university academic or other experienced colleagues within your department or organization who could work with you to carry out the analysis.

As we saw above, the utility of qualitative methods should not be underestimated in the field of QoL research, and part of their richness comes from the approach to data analysis. The analysis of qualitative data aims to describe and illuminate peoples' perceptions and experiences of a situation, rather than test hypotheses or produce findings that are generalizable to whole populations. Consequently, a different approach to analysis is taken. Qualitative data analysis requires a high degree of familiarity and a thorough understanding of the content of your, typically textual, data. Qualitative data should undergo thematic analysis; a process where key themes are identified within and between all of the participants' responses and presented alongside supportive quotes from the data. Most qualitative methods of analysis have some relationship to Grounded Theory, although the Framework approach of Ritchie and Lewis (2005) is increasingly common in healthcare research.

Finally, the interpretation of your findings, whatever analysis you use, should be cautious. This is because there will always be aspects of someone's life that have not been captured by a measure or interview and it is sensible to think about what these could be and whether they are likely to influence their satisfaction with life and your findings. You should estimate what these variables might be from a close inspection of the content of any topic guide or QoL measure's that you have used and interrogate it for what may not have been included.

Summary

A variety of methods exist for the assessment of QoL. The choice of method depends on the purpose of the research and also on a number of practical considerations (for example, respondent burden, respondent communication skills, resources, etc.). Objective measures, such as QALYS, are ideally placed to provide policymakers with an indication of the relative economic merits of two treatments in relation to their impact on QoL, whereas qualitative methods are subjective and better placed to illuminate the individual's experience of QoL. Between these two poles are standardized quality of life measures, which offer a compromise by measuring an individual's QoL in a standardized way.

Qualitative approaches can be used when you are asking in-depth questions about a client's or a group of clients' QoL experience. Alternatively, case study, cross sectional and comparative designs are well suited to quantitative methods of developing QoL evidence that describe and/or compare life quality from an individual to group level. Data collection relies on differing levels of communication skills and some methods may not be suitable or will require modification for certain clients.

Generating QoL evidence also lends itself to differing levels of analysis. In particular, quantitative designs can be analyzed and reported usefully through descriptive statistics or within more complicated designs using inferential, even multivariate, statistical analyses. However, when using statistical analyses to generate QoL evidence it is worthwhile remembering the client-centred role of QoL measurement and Bowling's (2001) conclusion that the individual might not feel how the statistics imply they should.

In summary, the key points for a clinician to consider when generating QoL evidence in the clinic are: the definition of QoL to be used, the variety of potential approaches to its measurement, and some of the implications they have for the client and the data collected. Finally, there is the need to understand the nature of QoL measurement development so that the use of such measures can be maximized to provide scientifically rigorous findings.

With all of these things in place, you should be ready to share your findings and make a difference.

References

Bowling, A. (2001) *Measuring Disease: A Review of Disease Specific Quality of Life Measurement Scales*. UK: Open University Press.

Connor, N. P., Cohen, S. B., Theis, S. M., Thibeault, S. L., Heatley, D. G., & Bless, D. M. (2008) Attitudes of children with dysphonia. *Journal of Voice* **22:2**, 197–209.

Eiser, C. & Morse, R. (2001) Quality-of-Life measures in chronic diseases of childhood. *Health Technology Assessment* **5:4**, 1–156.

Fayers, P. M. & Machin, D. (2007) *Quality of Life. The Assessment, Analysis and Interpretation of Patient-Reported Outcomes.* Chichester: John Wiley & Sons Ltd.

Hilari, K., Byng, S., Lamping, D., & Smith, S. C. (2003) Stroke and aphasia quality of life scale-39 (SAQOL-39). Evaluation of acceptability, reliability and validity. *Stroke* **34**, 1944–1950.

Klugman, T. M. & Ross, E. (2002) Perceptions of the impact of speech, language and hearing difficulties on quality of life of a group of South African persons with multiple sclerosis. *International Journal of Phoniatrics* **54:4**, 201–221.

Long, A. F., Hesketh, A., Paszek, G., Booth, M. & Bowen, A. (2008) Development of a reliable, self-report outcome measure for pragmatic trials of communication therapy following stroke: The Communication Outcome after Stroke (COAST) scale. *Clinical Rehabilitation* **22:12**, 1083–1094.

Markham, C., Van Laar, D., Gibbard, D., & Dean, T. (2009) Children with speech, language and communication needs: Their perceptions of their quality of life. *International Journal of Language and Communication Disorders* **44:5**, 1–21.

Ritchie, J. & Lewis, J. (2005) *Qualitative Research Practice: A Guide for Social Science Students Researchers.* London: Sage.

Wolfensberger, W. (1994) Let's hang up 'Quality of Life' as a hopeless term. In D. Goode (Ed.) *Quality of Life for Persons with Disabilities: International Perspectives and Issues.* Cambridge: Brookline Books.

World Health Organisation (1947) *World Health Organisation Constitution.* Retrieved from http://www.searo.who.int/LinkFiles/About_SEARO_const.pdf

World Health Organisation QOL Group (1993) *Measuring Quality of Life: The Developments of the World Health Organisation Quality of Life Instrument (WHOQOL).* Geneva: World Health Organisation.

World Health Organisation (2002) *International Classification of Functioning, Disability and Health.* Geneva: World Health Organisation.

Further reading

Cummins, R. A. (1997) Self-rated Quality of Life scales for people with an intellectual disability: A review. *Journal of Applied Research in Intellectual Disabilities* **10:3**, 199–216.

Rapley, M. (2003) *Quality of Life Research: A Critical Introduction.* London: Sage.

Roulstone, S. & McLeod, S. (Eds) (2011) *Listening to Children and Young People with Speech, Language and Communication Needs.* Guildford: J&R Press Ltd.

Resources

Patient-Reported Outcome and Quality of Life Instruments Database (PROQOLID) website, a database of QoL measures according to pathology and or population: http://www.proqolid.org/

6 The perspectives of others: What do people think of speech and language intervention and services?

Steven Bloch and Wendy Best

Learning outcomes

By the end of this chapter, you will be able to:

- Identify key reasons for seeking others' views
- Understand the main methods through which views can be sought
- Recognize the main challenges to seeking views
- Know where to go for further information and support

Introduction

In this chapter, we explore how to seek the views of others (so-called 'stakeholders') about our interventions and services. The views of clients and family members are particularly important to us but we may also include other professionals. Drawing on examples from developmental and acquired communication disorder settings, we provide a practical overview of local speech and language therapy (SLT) evaluation, the practicalities of obtaining users' views and how to use the information once collected.

Why do we need to understand the views of others?

It might seem odd to be thinking about the views of others when we could be clear in our own minds about the interventions and services we want to provide. With a little more money and some extra time, most speech and language therapists could outline a perfect service to meet everyone's needs. The reality, of course, is somewhat different. There are several reasons why listening to and understanding the views of others are now integral to national and local policy making (Department of Health, 2008):

- To evaluate intervention (for example, asking parents if they feel therapy has made a positive difference to their child's communication).

- To improve the overall service we offer (for example, establishing clients' experiences when admitted to a stroke unit).

- To reduce any mismatch between the expectations of others and what we can, are able or want to provide (for example, hospital nursing staff who ask us to manage all feeding as well as swallowing problems).

- To avoid the risk that we think we know best without ever considering the perspectives of others (especially those with severe communication difficulties who benefit from the provision of choices to express their views).

- To help promote our services to ensure they are understood by managers, other professionals and those responsible for commissioning or purchasing SLT services (for example, to present to head teachers and inclusion managers about the views of children and teachers on SLT).

- To help build confidence and trust between service users and providers.

- To show that we are listening to and acting on service users' concerns and complaints.

- To provide evidence for what many of us know; that we're already doing a good job but that some areas can always be improved upon.

What is so important about Speech and Language Therapy service users?

Listening, understanding and responding to the views of service users are now established practices in healthcare. All NHS organizations in England, for example, are now required to conduct postal surveys asking patients for their views on recent health service experiences. In addition, the Department of Health (2009) recognizes the need to ensure that '*Particular consideration should be given to gaining the participation of different groups, and any issues associated with those groups*' (p. 14). It is unusual, however, for audit managers to have the knowledge or experience to address all of the issues associated with people with communication disabilities, particularly those with complex needs. Such issues include the accessibility of existing service feedback mechanisms such as questionnaires or participation in focus groups. Speech and language therapists recognize the uniqueness of their service users and are well placed to ensure that the participation requirements of people with communication disabilities are appropriately promoted and managed.

What are the clinical issues?

The clinical issues that might prompt us to seek views of others can vary considerably. The following are selected examples:

- Introducing a new therapy technique: does it meet the needs of service users and is it practical? A new technique may have been shown to be effective in clinical trials but it might not necessarily be successful if there are local constraints or if it only makes small improvements to functional communication.

- Changing the ways in which a service is organized or delivered: patients with voice disorders, for example, might prefer the option of appointments out of normal working hours. You might want to establish whether this is the case by asking for feedback on clinic opening times.

- Problems with attendance and/or compliance: understanding why there is a problem and what will increase service uptake.

- Problems with adherence to programmes by others (for example, care staff following dysphagia advice in a nursing home or teaching assistants providing an agreed record of language activities carried out with a group).

Whose perspectives are we interested in?

Others in this context are commonly referred to as 'stakeholders'. A stakeholder could be an individual, group or organization with some level of interest in your treatment or service. This includes those who use your services as well as those involved in its planning and delivery. Typically, but not exclusively, the range of stakeholders involved in a SLT service includes those outlined in Figure 6.1.

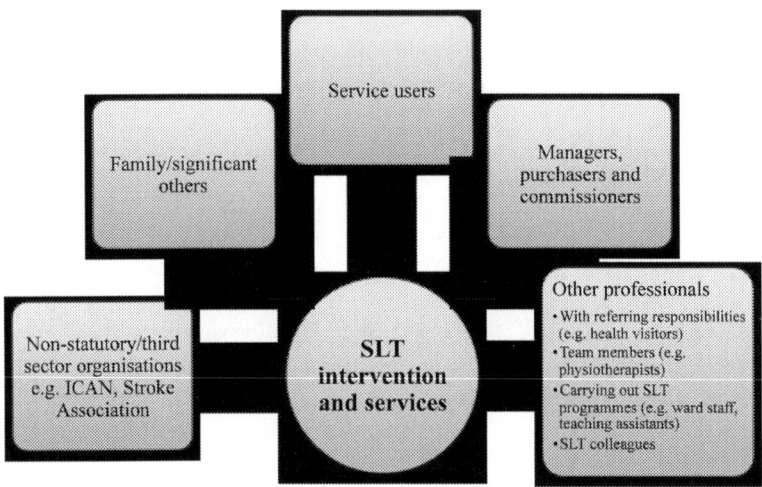

Figure 6.1 Speech and language therapy intervention and service stakeholders.

The list of stakeholders will vary depending on what you want to achieve. Seeking the views of service users alone could be enough if you want to establish the value of a particular intervention to them. You may, however, want to establish the views of service purchasers and commissioners if you are looking to establish how your services are perceived in comparison with other therapy services.

What do we already know about it?

An important issue is to ensure that your research question has not already been answered elsewhere. As our profession focuses increasingly on the evidence base for practice, and in particular in seeking practice-based evidence, it is important not to reinvent the wheel. For some areas this may be quite a simple process. The overall effectiveness of a particular treatment, for example, is likely to be reported in the clinical journals and through publically-available online research databases such as PubMed or Medline. We also acknowledge, however, that many SLT interventions and service delivery issues are not evidence based to peer review standard, and literature relating to user perspectives in the area you want to investigate could be relatively limited. In these cases, you may want to discuss your question with other SLTs, via specific interest groups, specialist advisors or through the Royal College of Speech and Language Therapists *Bulletin* 'any questions' page. Equally, many questions may be based on your own unique circumstances, including questions about a specific location or team service.

A range of views on SLT intervention and services has already been examined through a number of methods. Published studies relating specifically to the views of clients, parents and professionals include: the use of patient and clinician *focus groups* to inform the direction of aphasia services in Scotland (Law, Huby, Irving, Pringle, Conochie, Haworth, & Burston, 2010); *in-depth interviews* with children regarding their views of SLT in schools (Owen, Hayett, & Roulstone, 2004) and parents on their perceptions of service provision for their children with language needs (Dockrell & Lindsay, 2004), and finally *questionnaires* to establish the SLT expectations of people with Parkinson's disease and their carers (Miller, Noble, Jones, Deane, & Gibb, 2011), and parents' priorities for AAC intervention for their children (Calculator & Black, 2010). Many other examples can be found across most SLT clinical groups and environments.

In addition to published peer-reviewed evidence, a number of practical resources are also available. These are designed to either seek the views and experiences of general health service users or specifically to assist and promote engagement with people with communication disabilities (see Further Reading). These include the Talk for Scotland Toolkit and Connect's Communication Access (see Resources at the end of this chapter). Finally, the Royal College of Speech and Language Therapists' monthly *Bulletin* frequently includes highly accessible and practical features that incorporate the views of stakeholders.

Overall, there is plenty of evidence to show how stakeholders are involved in SLT service evaluation and treatment reviews. A thorough literature search will help identify those most relevant to your particular enquiry. We know that it is possible to elicit the views of stakeholders and that there are various methods for achieving this. These methods are discussed in the next section.

Refining the question

As therapists investigating the views of others, the big questions are whether our work is perceived as effective and whether we are providing the optimum service, be this the optimum therapy approach for pre-schoolers with dyspraxia for example, or the most appropriate multidisciplinary service to adults with progressive conditions living in the community.

In research, the more we think about and refine our question, the more useful the data will be that we obtain. Starting with local issues will automatically scale down the larger question and make the focus our individual service and the needs of our clients. Larger-scale implications might be appropriate but our initial focus will be local services. It is often useful to have an overarching question (for example, how do parents of Key Stage 1 children view the language resource base?), with specific sub-questions (for example, do parents find the information sent home too much or too little; would they prefer an alternative to a home-school book?). What is most useful is identifying questions, the answers to which can best inform our understanding and, where appropriate, inform realistic changes in our provision.

Whilst it may not be easy to involve service users at all stages of service evaluation and/or development, there is clear justification for eliciting their input whenever possible. Evidence indicates that questions seeking health service user feedback through surveys are often designed by managers and researchers rather than service users. It is important that service users and wider stakeholders are involved in the planning of your evaluation as well as its delivery, analysis and dissemination. This collaborative work can make a significant difference to the areas you cover and the subsequent impact that any changes will make. As a result, patient and public involvement (PPI) is now embedded within service evaluation and research activity.

In the next section we review the range of methods you might use in exploring the views of others.

What methods will I need to answer my question?

In this section, we provide a brief overview of the range of methods that are available to seek the views of others. The method(s) you use will depend on the research question you are asking, how many people you want to ask, their individual abilities and how long you have to analyze the answers to your questions. In our experience, it is always better to start off with a small, practical question that is likely to lead to a clear answer that has a direct bearing on our interventions/services.

It is also important, at this early stage, to consider whether your findings will need statistical analysis. Discussion about statistical analysis should take place at the start of the work rather than following data collection, as this is likely to inform the collection of views. For some smaller investigations, however, summaries without statistical analysis, beyond perhaps descriptive statistics such as average scores (mean, mode) and ranges, usually suffice. However, for a larger-scale quantitative evaluation advice from more experienced researchers or statisticians should be sought. For example, in a project with a large sample, statistical tests might be appropriate to compare views pre and post a change in service provision.

Additional time and support will often be required when seeking the views of people with communication disabilities but, in addition, establishing the views of people with profound learning or cognitive disabilities also needs careful consideration (see Further Reading). Ideally, one should discuss the accessibility of information with service users during the planning stages. This way, you have a much better chance of ensuring that your target group will be able to participate. We expand on this below.

Quantitative and qualitative methods (see Chapter 2) play an important role in informing our understanding of views of our services/interventions. It is perfectly possible, and often desirable, to use both for a clinically-based evaluation. For example, the effects of a block of therapy focusing on comprehension monitoring could be evaluated quantitatively in a specific task, such as how often clarification is requested in a small group setting. However, it could also be evaluated qualitatively, through asking teachers how they feel the therapy has impacted on children's understanding of language in the classroom. The boundaries between routine clinical practice and additional evaluation of stakeholders' views can blur. The difference, in the end, could be in the planning, the amount of evaluation and what is done with the information collected.

The following sections provide a brief overview of the most common methods for investigating people's perspectives, either for a research study or a service evaluation. They can be used individually or in combination as required.

Focus groups

A focus group is an informal meeting to discuss people's views and ideas about a specific topic, problem or experience. It should be organized to allow for flexibility and responsiveness to the needs of the individuals involved, comprising approximately six to twelve people with one or two facilitators. It should last no more than two hours and include a break for refreshments. Evidence suggests that focus groups can be a practical way of collecting information and informing health service delivery even in groups that may initially appear challenging, such as those from mixed cultural or linguistic backgrounds (Halcomb, Gholizadeh, DiGiacomo, Phillips, & Davidson, 2007). The representativeness of a focus group needs careful planning and one needs to be aware of how agreements are reached in a group of individuals who may share a common diagnosis or disorder, but who possibly have very different perspectives and experiences. The results can be used to generate ideas for more detailed follow-up, for example, through a survey or questionnaire.

Practical tips

- Involve stakeholders in planning the group.
- Clarify the purpose and objectives of the group with everyone involved in advance.
- Make sure the venue is accessible to all participants. If transport is required, make sure this is organized in good time.
- Invite an experienced facilitator. It may be helpful to ask a colleague or manager to facilitate a group if you have a strong interest in the outcomes.
- Agree ground rules and an agenda for the group.
- If one individual takes over, then consider strategies for harnessing his/her enthusiasm such as chairing a sub-group or assisting others to communicate.
- Ensure the main points of any discussion are recorded, either by an audio-recording device such as a digital voice recorder or handwritten notes. Arrange a note taker in advance if required.
- Use prepared questions and themes relating to the topic(s) for discussion.

- Write up any thoughts or observations immediately after the meeting.
- Feedback outcomes to the group as soon as possible.

Surveys/questionnaires

Questionnaires are relatively straightforward to administer and can be used to obtain views, experiences and levels of satisfaction. They are also useful for measuring baseline information and to evaluate change over time, for example to compare views before and after a change in service provision. Using appropriate language and/or visual representations, the content and presentation of questionnaires can be adapted to match the cognitive and linguistic abilities of the intended sample. The main challenge in using questionnaires is in avoiding bias or ambiguity in the questions. It is always a good idea to involve stakeholders in designing the questions and then to pilot your questionnaire on a small number of the study population first, allowing plenty of time for re-drafting as required.

Care needs to be taken to not ask questions that might raise unrealistic expectations. For example, there is little value in asking your local Parkinson's disease self-help group if they would like access to an intensive speech intelligibility treatment programme if there is no chance of you being able to provide it. Instead, consider the range of interventions you *can* realistically provide within the resources available and then seek input on the group's preferences, priorities and previous experiences. Service user feedback should not just be used as a lobbying tool for more resources although clearly it can be used as evidence to support requests for resource reviews and allocations.

Practical tips

- Be clear about what you are trying to accomplish, what you want the information for and how you will use the results

- Avoid bias in your questions by phrasing them as neutrally as possible. Discuss your first draft questions with colleagues to help you refine the wording of your questions

- Structure questions carefully; consider the balance between multiple choice and free text questions.

- Keep it short; ideally a questionnaire should take no more than 5–10 minutes to complete.

- Always pilot the questionnaire with a small group of the people whose views and ideas you want.

- Think about how you will reach your target group. If posting, include a freepost or stamped addressed envelope for returns.

- Online questionnaire tools can be a relatively efficient way of gathering data but might require more design work, particularly if symbols and pictures are required.

- There is still a substantial proportion of the population without regular access to the Internet, in particular older people who are the heaviest users of health services.

Interviews

In-depth (semi-structured) one-to-one interviews are used to collect qualitative data. They aim to understand the respondent's point of view, experiences and needs rather than make generalizations. The interviewer can explore areas more deeply and ask for the reasons behind responses. Interviews are, however, more time consuming to conduct and analyze than surveys. The interviewer needs to provide opportunities for the respondent to explore his or her own views and experiences whilst ensuring the overall aims of the interview are met.

Practical tips

- Decide what it is you want from the interviews first and how you plan to analyze the responses.

- Discuss the areas you want to explore with stakeholders and colleagues before you finalise the main interview question areas.

- Draw up a topic guide to ensure you cover all of the areas of interest to you.

- If your service users have significant communication, learning and/or cognitive disabilities, ensure the questions you ask are presented in an appropriate way and that the interviewee is able to respond. Your PPI group can help you with this.

- Decide how you will record the interview responses.

- Use open-ended questions. Some will be planned (*'Tell me about...'*) and some will arise naturally during the interview (*'You said a moment ago...'*, *'Can you tell me more...?'*).

- Clarify what is being said so there are no misunderstandings.

- Aim for a conversational feel: questions should be asked when it feels appropriate; they may be planned or spontaneous.

- The wording of the questions may vary in different interviews. This is acceptable as long as the main areas are covered in each interview.

- Consider using an interviewer who is external to the topic or service being discussed.

- Keep the number of interviews manageable; many improvement ideas can come from just a few interviews.

Other methods for seeking views and experiences are available, including observation (shadowing), diaries, web groups and online forums. Further advice on choosing the right research methods in health service evaluation research can be found at the Picker Institute website (see Table 6.1 and additional on-line resources below).

Further discussion regarding the strengths and weakness of all of the feedback methods mentioned here can be found in Coulter, Fitzpatrick and Cornwell (2009).

Table 6.1 Choosing the right research methods (Picker Institute Europe, 2009).

Task	Suggested research method
Monitoring performance and assessing quality	Patient experience surveys
Determining priorities of the local population	Population surveys
Ongoing engagement	Patient panels
Identifying issues of concern to key stakeholders	Analysis of written materials
In depth investigation of attitudes and beliefs	Focus groups Interviews
Testing services	Observation in healthcare settings

Getting into the detail

As with your clinical intervention, gathering, analyzing and acting on the views of others is, ultimately, a practical task. It should always begin with clear goals about the information you want, and end with some form of evaluation to measure the impact of any changes you have made.

How do we identify the stakeholders?

There are two straightforward stages involved in identifying your stakeholders:

1. Decide which *group(s)* of stakeholders you are interesting in listening to (see Figure 6.1 above). This will often be service users but clearly this will depend on what you want to find out.

2. Decide which *individuals* within the group(s) you want to involve. This may be highly specific, such as parents of children with cochlear implants, or more general, for example, anyone who has attended the SLT outpatient clinic at a local hospital over the last six months.

How do we get a representative sample of views?

As with any sampling, responses are likely to be forthcoming from those with the most interest and those most able to engage in the process. Facilitating the participation of people who are less likely, or able, to take part may be challenging but is particularly important given the risk of exclusion faced by many of the people we work with. The potential challenges we need to consider here include:

- The effects of any communication impairment on the ability to engage with consultation

- Cultural distinctions

- Physical, mobility and/or sensory impairments

- Small sample pools; for example, the number of people with a specific condition within your health care or education area

On paper, these do not appear too problematic, but in reality we all recognize how hard it can be to ensure a full range of views is elicited, particularly where service users are involved. It is important to be aware of the challenges and consider how best to mitigate their impact. The effects of many communication impairments can, for example, be dealt with through advanced planning, discussion and support. Making sure there is an established mechanism for the expression of preferences or choices could be helpful here. If physical or travel restrictions make it too hard to arrange a focus group, then it is worth considering the use of email, web groups and/or services like Skype.

Gaining feedback from community or self-help meetings can be very efficient but remember that not everyone is able, or wants, to attend such groups. Try to balance your sample between those who are clearly able and motivated to participate with those who are, for whatever reason, disengaged from community participation.

Small sample pools should not be problematic for local service feedback. If you have a caseload of three people with Huntington's disease, or three families whose children have had cochlear implants, for example, then it is acceptable to either elicit the views from all three or to consider linking up with other clinicians to widen the sample as required.

Are there any specific ethical issues?

It is likely that many of the ideas described in this chapter will be classed as audit or service evaluation rather than research and therefore not subject to formal ethical review. Local research and development officers can provide guidance on this, particularly when you are working with vulnerable children or adults. If you have any doubts, then contact your local research governance or ethics committee for advice. Details of local UK NHS health ethics committees can be found online (see Resources).

With reference to service-user views and feedback, the main ethical issues that are likely to arise relate to confidentiality, emotional distress and clinical care. SLTs are used to respecting confidentiality, but when collecting and reporting on the views of service users it can be easy to forget the importance of data protection and information storage. Anyone involved in your feedback work needs to know what you will be doing with that information, where it will be stored, for how long and whether or not confidential details such as names will be kept alongside feedback.

Emotional distress in research can arise as an ethical issue if service users have experienced problematic care on which they are then asked to feedback. This is best managed by ensuring that participants know how to contact you and/or access support services if the process of feedback leads to distress.

The ethical issue of clinical care should be acknowledged. If you ask your service users to feedback or evaluate your own service, or even that of colleagues, then there may be a perception that anything critical or negative could affect subsequent care or professional relationships. You need to make the point, as clearly as possible, that nothing your participants say will affect their current or future healthcare. Such an explanation is a requirement for NHS ethics approval, but for service users with communication needs you may need to consider how to get this information across, beyond a standard patient information sheet.

What kinds of data should we collect?

Whether you are interested in receiving views about the pre-school clinic waiting list system or the long-term outcomes of the nursing home staff training package, one important distinction is between establishing people's levels of satisfaction and their experience. Instead of asking service users to feedback their level of satisfaction with a service or treatment (e.g. on a scale ranging from excellent to very poor), they might be asked to report their experience of, for example, whether certain events took place during an episode of care. These types of questions are intended to elicit reports on what actually occurred, rather than the patient's *evaluation* of what occurred (Coulter et al., 2009). This avoids the problem of positive responses that commonly arise when service users are asked to rate a service, particularly when they have just received that service or are being asked directly by the clinician involved in their therapy.

When should we collect the data?

Real-time patient feedback through new technologies is highly visible in the current NHS, but local practical issues and resources are likely to dictate the methods and timing of your feedback collection. If you are running a training session for teachers, then it seems sensible to collect questionnaire format feedback on their views immediately after the event; collecting views prior to the event may also be desirable if you are seeking to evaluate the effects of your training (see Chapter 7). However, there are instances where delaying the collection of feedback could be advantageous; for example, asking a patient to comment on your swallowing treatment as they are discharged from hospital could yield a different response if they are asked two weeks later. There are no rules dictating the timing and it may well depend on your opportunities for data collection and/or how quickly you want to act on the feedback. If it is not feasible to delay feedback collection, then asking for both positive and negative or critical comments is useful in ensuring a balanced feedback profile. This can be achieved, for example, by asking for at least three things that work well and three things that could be improved.

Who should collect the data?

In many cases, stakeholder views will be sought by the clinician(s) involved in the service delivery. This makes sense given that they will already know how their service is provided and what the key issues are likely to be. However, consideration should be given to who collects the data itself. Coulter et al. (2009) comment that 'on-site' surveys in hospitals often rely on staff inviting patients to respond, running the risk that they will elicit only favourable comments. For a more realistic picture, it may be better if data collection can be organized by a non-staff member such as an assistant, volunteer or even a SLT student.

Should we collaborate with others?

Collecting data and acting on findings can be accomplished by an individual clinician, but might be easier when done as part of a larger team or group. Small-scale feedback may be best suited to an individual's caseload or, in some cases, a particular client group. For the latter, you might want to investigate whether other clinicians are interested in working with you. Specific interest groups (SIGs) are an ideal vehicle for collaboration with others, who are likely to share common clinical interests and experiences. In addition, you might want to look outside of SLT and consider collecting views jointly with other professionals, particularly those with a shared interest in, for example, child development or stroke rehabilitation. Thinking together about evaluation of provision across boundaries, for example, health and education, is likely to be appropriate at managerial level and is more likely to facilitate integrated care from the user's viewpoint.

At a more general level, many health and education organizations have existing mechanisms for feedback. These mechanisms include managers responsible for audit, data collection design and implementation. Establishing links with these managers is one good way in which to learn about the existing processes already in place for service user involvement.

How can we embed data-gathering into our everyday clinical work?

Whilst it may be beneficial to carry out a feedback exercise as an entirely separate activity, there is also a variety of ways in which you can collect service user views as part of your everyday clinical work. One straightforward way is to extend your routine meetings with others to seek their views more formally. Examples include:

- if your team currently has SEN meetings with local educational psychologists, you may be able to schedule 15 minutes at the end to seek views on SLT contributions to the statementing process;

- if you are running a group for people with Parkinson's disease, you may be able to organize a parallel focus group for carers to explore their perceptions of SLT.

Short surveys and/or questionnaires seeking feedback on treatment can also be arranged as part of your clinical routine. Service users and significant others can be asked questions in person at the end of their treatment or via post or email (see above on the timing of feedback). For more general feedback on service delivery, it might be possible to have a feedback or ideas box in a waiting room area. By repeating a process either annually or at points of change, it is possible to compare data over time and to consider the effects of any changes you have made to treatments or service delivery.

Analysis

> Inadequate analysis, leading to poor presentation of the results, is the surest way to ensure that patient views have little or no impact. When placed alongside the results of clinical trials and major observational studies, it is essential that patient feedback is rigorously analyzed and the messages clearly presented. It can be all too easy to dismiss the information as 'simply anecdotal' when it should be seen as a crucial and equal partner to data on safety and effectiveness.
>
> (Department of Health, 2009: p. 20)

Having gathered your clients' views you are now ready to make sense of what they have said. Analysis need not be complicated and will vary with the method of collection. Once again, we would caution that any statistical analysis of the data needs to be planned alongside the development of your question.

Analysis involves making sense of your findings. Different research methods lend themselves to different forms of analysis, but you should be providing intelligible and clear results based on the information and feedback you have received. To do this, you need to be able to present the results of your research in a way that makes sense to you as well as others.

To cite an example of our own, in a recent study of residential home service user views (Bloch & Maxim, 2010), 70 people with varying degrees of communication disability were interviewed. The interviews were video recorded and then analyzed in two ways. First, a *quantitative* analysis was undertaken, involving coding answers to give them a numerical value. For example, for the question 'Do you understand printed notices and messages here at your home?' codes were generated for: yes, no and sometimes. This meant that a simple descriptive average (mean) could be provided: 33% of respondents said 'no'. A *qualitative* analysis was used for answers that could not easily be coded such as 'Why are you unable to take part in activities here at home?' Using template analysis (King, 2004) all of the comments were reviewed and were then grouped into five main themes. Comments were then allocated to the themes according to whether they were negative or positive. This then enabled the researchers to view all of the comments and judge the overall balance of views as well as those voiced most frequently. This type of analysis is not complex, but does demand time, a methodical approach and discussion to ensure the results are being analyzed fairly and reliably.

What if someone complains about our service or intervention?

Service users who have been asked to comment on the treatment they receive may wish to make a complaint; either about your own service or that provided by another organization. If this does happen, then you need to be able to explain your organization's complaints procedure and/or ensure the service user has adequate support to manage any resulting anxiety or problems arising from the disclosure. Whilst any service/treatment feedback data collected should be confidential, you still have an ethical and professional responsibility to manage problems in line with national and local guidelines and regulations.

An opportunity to provide feedback can generate criticisms of services and individuals. Whilst the person giving this feedback might not ever want to make a formal complaint, they should be aware of the mechanisms of how to do so. If your evaluation work is part of a formal NHS ethically approved study, then an explanation of how to complain will be in your participant information sheet. If your evaluation is a local audit then you still need to consider how service users can be informed about complaints procedures.

Feedback, dissemination and closing the loop

> Collecting feedback by itself has no value. It needs to help clinical and management teams to identify aspects of their service that need to improve, so the team can take appropriate action.

(Department of Health, 2009: p. 12)

Once the views of your stakeholders have been collected and the results analyzed you are in a position to take action. The specific actions you take will depend on a number of factors but there are at least three processes to accomplish: feedback, dissemination (see Chapter 9) and closing the loop.

Sharing your findings with those who have contributed ensures that those who have participated in your research see the purpose of your work and feel part of its development. It also increases the chances of further participation in any future view-seeking exercises. Participant feedback need not be a complex procedure but should be relevant, balanced, accessible and timely. For service users in particular, it is vital that any feedback is presented in a concise and clear format that matches the communication abilities of those who have shared their views. People with communication disabilities may require feedback presented in a format using symbols or multimedia. Further, it might need to be presented verbally/interactively rather than, or as well as, in print. The principles mentioned throughout this chapter, and in Chapter 9, should be followed to ensure that communication is facilitated as required.

How do we close the loop?

As well as ensuring that findings are fed back to those involved in providing their views and then disseminated to the various relevant stakeholders, it might be necessary to make changes. This is called 'closing the loop'. The results of your research should show you where things are working well and where changes can be made. If the feedback points to a large number of changes, then it will be necessary to prioritize. Prioritization here means selecting those areas that you feel can be improved, within the resources available, and which will make a difference. It is advisable to involve your stakeholders in this process through discussion. To avoid unrealistic expectations, you need to be honest about what is feasible. This will mean that service users and others have a more realistic understanding about how change can work and why, for example, an increase in the number of therapists might not be possible in the short term, given the need for wider health/education business planning.

Any changes you do make should be well documented and the effects measured. These can then be fed back to stakeholders to show how their involvement has led to treatment and/or overall service improvements. Whilst there is very little published evidence showing the direct impact of feedback on SLT service development, a number of clinicians contacted by the authors do report such improvements. At one teaching hospital, for example, people with memory problems reported needing an appointment reminder closer to the actual appointment than currently provided. As a result, the hospital has started an automated text messaging service trial to remind patients of their outpatient appointments. This has helped reduce missed appointment rates. At a children's hospital, an audit of parent satisfaction led to the provision of a play worker to look after the children whilst the parents spoke to the diagnostic team. Clinicians found this interesting, as received clinical wisdom was that parents should have their children present whilst diagnoses are being discussed. In truth, the majority of parents were clear: they did not want to have to look after their children whilst trying to listen to important information. A final example is drawn from a local authority's pre-school teaching team. Their survey explored the views and needs of parents of children with complex needs. This resulted in funding for a multidisciplinary team providing an additional 1–2 hours a week, supporting children with social communication difficulties. A follow-up parent questionnaire identified a need for more SLT input leading to the provision of SLT groups.

Conclusions

Investigating what others think of your SLT intervention and/or provision is an integral element of service development. Taken together with clinical evidence, guidelines and local priorities, the views and experiences of others help you to understand how your service is perceived and the degree to which it meets the needs of your service users.

Asking what others think about your intervention and service need not be complex or costly, but it does require careful planning. Of particular importance is the recognition that people with communication disabilities need time and support to fully express their views. The demands this could make should not be underestimated.

Speech and language therapists are ideally placed to ensure that the views of people with communication needs and other stakeholders are understood. Evolving your interventions for the benefit of your service users is a natural outcome of this process.

Summary

This chapter has highlighted the importance of seeking the views of others as this is integral to making improvements to your service. The views of SLT service users in particular need to be considered and, indeed, stakeholders can be involved in how you evaluate your intervention and services right from the start of the process. To have maximum impact, it is important that the questions you ask should be relevant to you and the people who use your service. There are a range of quantitative and qualitative methods that are suitable for eliciting the views of people with communication disabilities, including focus groups, questionnaires and interviews. Findings should be analyzed in a way that makes sense to you and to those whose views you sought. Moreover, they should be fed back to those involved in the data collection and disseminated to interested stakeholders. The aim is to 'close the loop' by taking action and making changes wherever possible.

Acknowledgements

We are extremely grateful to Pam Czerniewska, Julia Johnson and Katie Price for their examples from clinical practice and the Picker Institute Europe for their kind permission to use materials from their online patient feedback resource.

References

Bloch, S. & Maxim, J. (2010) Evaluation of the Leonard Cheshire Disability Communication Project – Final report. London: University College London.

Calculator, S. N. & Black, T. (2010) Parents' priorities for AAC and related instruction for their children with Angelman Syndrome. *Augmentative and Alternative Communication* **26:1**, 30–40.

Coulter, A., Fitzpatrick, R., & Cornwell, J. (2009) *The Point of Care: Measuring Patients' Experience in Hospital*. London: The King's Fund.

Department of Health (2008) *High Quality Care for All*. London: Department of Health.

Department of Health (2009) *Understanding What Matters: A Guide to Using Patient Feedback to Transform Services*. London: Department of Health.

Dockrell, J. E. & Lindsay, G. (2004) Whose job is it? Parents' concerns about the needs of their children with language problems. *Journal of Special Education* **37:4**, 225–235.

Halcomb, E. J., Gholizadeh, L., DiGiacomo M., Phillips, J., & Davidson, P. M. (2007) Literature review: Considerations in undertaking focus group research with culturally and linguistically diverse groups. *Journal of Clinical Nursing* **16:6**, 1000–1011.

King, N. (2004) Using templates in the thematic analysis of texts. In C. Cassell & G. Symon. (Eds) *Essential Guide to Qualitative Research in Organizational Research*. London: Sage, pp. 256–270.

Law, J., Huby, G., Irving, A. M., Pringle, A. M., Conochie, D., Haworth, C., & Burston, A. (2010) Reconciling the perspective of practitioner and service user: Findings from The Aphasia in Scotland study. *International Journal of Language and Communication Disorders* **45:5**, 551–560.

Miller, N., Noble, E., Jones, D., Deane, K. H., & Gibb, C. (2011) Survey of speech and language therapy provision for people with Parkinson's disease in the United Kingdom: Patients' and carers' perspectives. *International Journal of Language & Communication Disorders* **46:2**, 179–188.

Owen, R., Hayett, L., & Roulstone, S. (2004) Children's views of speech and language therapy in school: Consulting children with communication difficulties. *Child Language Teaching and Therapy* **20:1**, 55–73.

Picker Institute Europe (2009) *Using Patient Feedback: A Practical Guide to Improving Patient Experience*. Oxford: Picker Institute.

Further reading

Boynton, P. M. (2004) Administering, analysing, and reporting your questionnaire. *British Medical Journal* **328:7452**, 1372 –1375.

Boynton, P. M. & Greenhalgh, T. (2004) Selecting, designing, and developing your questionnaire. *British Medical Journal* **328:7451**, 1312–1315.

Brewster, S. J. (2004) Putting words into their mouths? Interviewing people with learning disabilties and little/no speech. *British Journal of Learning Disabilities* **32:4**, 166–169.

Carlsson, E., Paterson, B. L., Scott-Findlay, S., Ehnfors, M., & Ehrenberg, A. (2007) Methodological issues in interviews involving people with communication impairments after acquired brain damage. *Qualitative Health Research* **17:10**, 1361–1371.

Gillham, B. (2010) *Developing a Questionnaire*. London: Continuum.

Murphy, J., Tester, S., Hubbard, G., Downs, M., & MacDonald, C. (2005) Enabling frail older people with a communication difficulty to express their views: The use of Talking Mats as an interview tool. *Health and Social Care in the Community* **13:2**, 95–107.

Owens, J. S. (2006) Accessible information for people with complex communication needs. *Augmentative and Alternative Communication* **22:3**, 196–208.

Pring, T. (2005) *Research Methods in Communication Disorders*. London: Whurr.

Ware, J. (2004) Ascertaining the views of people with profound and multiple learning disabilities. *British Journal of Learning Disabilities* **32:4**, 175–179.

For a series of papers on the development of innovative ways of eliciting the views of children and young people with learning disabilities, see the *British Journal of Learning Disabilities*, 2004, volume 32, issue 4, edited by J. Porter and A. Lewis.

Resources

Communication Forum Scotland: Talk for Scotland toolkit for communication access:

http://www.communicationforumscotland.org.uk/2010/TK_Home.php

Connect: Toolkit for communication (aphasia) access: http://www.ukconnect.org/communicationaccess.aspx

Evaluation Trust: Evaluation methods toolkit:

http://www.evaluationtrust.org/tools/toolkit

INVOLVE: Supporting public involvement in NHS, public health and social care research

http://www.invo.org.uk/

NHS health ethics committees:

http://www.nres.npsa.nhs.uk/contacts/nres-committee-directory/

NHS Institute for Innovation and Improvement: Quality and Service Improvement Tools for Stakeholder Analysis:

http://www.institute.nhs.uk/quality_and_service_improvement_tools/quality_and_service_improvement_tools/stakeholder_analysis.html

Picker Institute Europe: Ways of examining patient views in healthcare:

http://www.pickereurope.org/

7 We are doing some training. What are the benefits?

Yvonne Wren

Learning outcomes

By the end of this chapter, you will be able to:

- Understand the importance of assessing the value and impact of training
- Know what is important to assess
- Know how findings can impact at a variety of levels – individual, organization, setting, home, future training and commissioning of training

---

Introduction

Providing training or professional development opportunities is an integral part of our role as speech and language therapists. Our audience varies depending upon our client group and specialist area but the key question following the delivery of any training is the same: has it made a difference?

The 'difference' we want to see will vary and will operate at different levels. In most cases, the audience for training will not be individuals with communication impairments or difficulties with feeding or swallowing, but their carers or a range of others who may work with or have some interaction with individuals with these needs. Whilst we are keen to see a change in participants' knowledge and skills, ultimately we want to be reassured that our training has had an impact on people with communication impairment or feeding and swallowing difficulties. We want to know that the time spent preparing and delivering a training package or professional development programme has resulted in tangible improvements for our clients and others with similar difficulties in terms of their progress, their everyday interactions and their general wellbeing.

This chapter explores the issues surrounding the delivery of training in the field of speech and language therapy. The focus is on how training can be evaluated and at what levels evaluation is possible. The chapter will use a published report of a training programme (Wren, 2003) to illustrate some of the issues involved but will also make reference to other types of training targeting a range of possible audiences. For simplicity, the chapter will use the term 'training' to cover a variety of activities including professional development and awareness-raising. As any training for individuals with communication impairment could be regarded as 'intervention', which is covered in Chapters 4 and 5, this chapter will focus on training for relatives, carers and other professionals.

The chapter will use the same format as others chapters in this section, focusing initially on the challenges we face as clinician researchers trying to evaluate the training we offer. The chapter will move on to discuss what is already known in the field before considering the issue of refining the research question in relation to course evaluations. Types of methodology which are appropriate to particular research questions are covered next, followed by a discussion of the types of methods of data collection and analysis that suit particular types of enquiry. The chapter concludes with a summary of the steps to consider at each stage in the evaluation of a training course.

What are the clinical issues or challenges?

In an environment where outcomes and cost effectiveness are the current drivers for services, there is a need to show that training delivers on both. This is the key challenge to anyone delivering and evaluating any sort of training. Without this evidence, future funding for your training programme could be reduced or cut altogether with consequences for your clients.

To effectively measure outcomes and cost effectiveness, it is essential to know what you are hoping to achieve through your training. Primary outcomes will vary but can broadly be grouped into one of the following:

- An increase in awareness

- The acquisition of new skills

- The acquisition of new knowledge

- Changes in behaviour

It is this last outcome which is the most crucial and which should occur as a result of a change in the first three. Without a change in the behaviour of those attending training, at some level, it is hard to justify the input in time, effort and money to plan and deliver the training. Yet this is the most difficult of the four to measure. Indeed, it has even been described as the 'holy grail' of inspectors and evaluators of training (Oldroyd & Hall, 1991).

Off-putting as this might seem, it is nevertheless possible to evaluate the outcomes of a training programme provided that you as the investigator are clear about what you are trying to measure and that you use the most appropriate methods to fit your inquiry. These issues are covered in more detail in the sections, 'Refining your question' and 'What methods will I need to answer my question?'.

Of vital importance, however, is the need to consider evaluation at the beginning when planning any training. There is a need for the aims and objectives to be clearly stated and defined in order that they can be measured. Moreover, in nearly all cases, there is a need to carry out pre- and post-training assessments to measure the outcomes and impact of the training.

Purpose of training

As speech and language therapists, we become involved in training others for a variety of purposes.

Working within a stroke unit setting, there could be a need for an ongoing programme for the multidisciplinary team on the types of communication impairment that people might experience. The broad purpose of the training might be to explain the nature and impact of these impairments and how best to communicate with patients during their work with them as physios, nurses, OTs, etc.

As a school-based SLT, you might run an INSET day or a series of twilight sessions for teachers and teaching assistants. These could be general awareness-raising sessions or a more detailed programme of training, for example to enable assistants to deliver SLT programmes. A real-life example of this style of training is described in Wren (2003) in which two school-based speech and language therapists evaluated the change in knowledge and skills of teachers and teacher assistants following attendance on a training programme consisting of one whole day and five twilight sessions.

In the community setting, the speech and language therapist working with nursery staff and children's centres could plan training to highlight the opportunities that everyday activities provide for language enrichment.

Whilst the examples above describe training other professionals, there is also a variety of training needs for carers and relations of individuals with communication impairment. Parents of children in the pre-school years might be offered a 'Hanen®' programme in which they learn how they can promote the language development of their children in the home. Relatives of individuals with aphasia might be offered an information session regarding what to expect and how best to hold a conversation with their loved one.

Style of presentation of training

The type of training which is designed and offered to participants will depend on the overall purpose, the potential audience and limitations such as time, money and locations.

Where the purpose of the training is to increase awareness and knowledge of a particular issue, a lecture-style presentation could be selected to introduce participants to the theory behind a subject in order to develop their knowledge and understanding. At the other extreme, if the aim of the training is to demonstrate a particular technique or strategy related to a particular client's needs, then the most effective approach could be a one-to-one coaching session with an assistant to or carer of the client.

Between these extremes is a whole variety of styles of presentation including workshops, use of role play and simulation techniques, case studies, group and individual exercises and group discussion. With advances in technology, there is a range of options to support training through the use of DVD and audio clips as well as video downloads from *YouTube*. In addition, online programmes can be developed which enable a course participant to access the training at a time and place to suit them. The usefulness of online methods extends to the development of self-appraisal tools to identify where the individual course participant needs to begin their training and, indeed, determine the distance travelled in their understanding and knowledge afterwards. While technology can therefore be used to assess knowledge of skills, it is not yet able to assess application of those skills, and in terms of identifying changes to behaviour, other methods such as video observations and peer appraisal would need to be applied.

What do we already know about it?

Searching the literature

The need to carry out a literature search and to critically appraise relevant papers is described in detail in Chapter 3, together with an explanation of how to do this. With regard to the topic of the current chapter, the kind of literature to explore will be that which describes the evaluation of other training programmes. Whilst the development of the training programme itself will no doubt have required some searching of papers and databases in order to ensure that current evidence-based practice is being disseminated and applied, the literature relating to evaluations of training programmes will help to illustrate ways in which evaluation can be carried out.

Literature searching in the area of evaluation of training should not be restricted to the speech and language field. Rather, a range of sources which fit with the client group whose needs ultimately you are trying to address should be sought. For example, if you are planning to evaluate a training package for early years practitioners, you might look for evaluations of other early years programmes provided by non-SLTs. Similarly, a programme aimed at increasing awareness of communication impairment in the elderly and delivered to staff in nursing homes could look for reports of evaluations of training for nursing home staff from other professionals such as dieticians. Exploring a broad range of sources will provide a more rounded and multidimensional picture of the issues relating to evaluation of training with the intended audience.

Typically, a range of methods will be reported depending on the specific question being asked and the nature of the training provided. Part of your appraisal of this literature will be to determine how closely a study, described in a paper, fits with your objectives and whether some of the methods might usefully be employed in your own plans. With the benefit of hindsight, you will be able to identify some of the disadvantages of the methods used and adapt an approach to suit your own needs.

When you know what type of methods you will be using for your evaluation, you might also want to search the literature for other examples of this. So if you plan on using a questionnaire to assess changes in confidence levels post training, you would want to search for reports of others who have used questionnaires to evaluate training in SLT or related fields. Alternatively, if the type of evaluation which best suits your need is a participant observation approach, then the literature relating to ethnographic methods, a qualitative approach which seeks to describe and understand the nature of those who are being studied, will be most useful.

In a similar way, it could be helpful to identify ways in which evaluations have been conducted with reference to the primary objective or presentation style used in your training programme. For example, you could explore evaluations of training packages that have been used for a range of audiences where the objective was to measure change in awareness and knowledge; or you might look for evaluations of workshop-style training packages in healthcare in general if this is the method of presentation you are going to evaluate.

Chapter 3 gives detailed advice regarding literature searching but you will have learned from this that using the most appropriate search terms is vital to retrieving the right papers. In terms of evaluating training, think of the range of words which could be substituted for evaluation – *measurement, assessment, appraisal* are just some. Moreover, use the abbreviated form with a wildcard, for example, 'evaluat*', in order to search for titles and abstracts with the words 'evaluate' or 'evaluation'. Similarly for training – other words that could be used include 'education', 'development', 'instruction' and 'teaching'.

Finally, remember to use the 'grey' literature as well – the reports and magazine articles which you won't find using database searches. Google and other search engines could help to reveal some of these but also look through recent paper copies of publications relevant to your participants, for example, *Nursing Times, Special Children,* and the *Times Educational Supplement,* and identify reports of similar activity within your workplace.

Other sources of information

Aside from the more formal literature searching, colleagues can also be a useful source of information. Local colleagues will have particular knowledge of the demographic and cultural makeup of the locality in which you are operating and will be able to offer opinions as to which types of method of evaluation might be most suitable and which could be alienating.

Colleagues from further afield but within the profession can be another useful source of advice. Discussing your plans with others who have reported evaluations using similar methods could be a useful way to identify possible pitfalls. Members of the multidisciplinary team might also be able to offer a unique perspective on plans for training and evaluation based on their own experience – either with the same audience or using the same methods.

Most importantly, however, is the need to consult with the training participants. To maximize the validity of your evaluation, you will need to ensure a response from a high number of participants. Post training, those participants who are most likely to comply with an evaluation will be those who feel the evaluation is asking the questions they want to answer. So it is essential to talk with participants at an early stage and understand what questions they have, what they hope to get out of the training and what changes they hope to see in themselves and others post training.

Ideally, this discussion should take place some time before the training event happens in order for the aims and objectives of the course participants to be incorporated into the plans for the CPD. In many cases, it may not be feasible to link in with all course participants but it should be possible to make contact with a representative of the participants, such as their manager or the person who has requested the training, to clarify what is required.

In many cases, but not always, the aims and objectives of the course participants will fit with the objectives identified by the course leader and/or the individual who has commissioned the training. In such a case, a maximum response from participants to an evaluation will be achieved when the method used to evaluate uncovers answers to their questions as well as your own.

In addition, it is necessary to gauge how participants feel about anonymity in a post-training evaluation. If the course leader is also the person carrying out the evaluation, attendees might feel less able to give negative feedback. Certain approaches to evaluation make this anonymity impossible, however, and may result in skewed findings. For example, one possibility for evaluating a training programme is to use an open-ended interview with course participants in which they are asked about changes to their behaviour post training. If the interviews are carried out by the course leader, participants might feel obliged to exaggerate the changes they have made in order to please their interviewer. If an alternative interviewer is used, participants may feel able to be more honest in their responses.

Refining the question

As mentioned in the title, the key question in any evaluation of training is 'Has it made a difference?' The next question is therefore, quite naturally, 'Difference to what?' The answer to this will depend on the motivations and drivers for the person carrying out the evaluation. If the main purpose of the evaluation is to justify the funding spent on the course for those who have commissioned it, then issues relating to cost effectiveness as well as what difference the training has made for your clients will be paramount.

With regard to refining your question, Guskey (2000) provides a useful hierarchy of outcomes of training which is helpful in identifying what difference we want to measure. He identifies five levels of outcomes which might be considered in an evaluation of training:

- Participants' reaction
- Participants' learning
- Organization support and change
- Participants' use of new knowledge and skills
- Student learning outcomes

Guskey was writing specifically in the context of education and his 'student learning outcomes' therefore relate to changes to school children in response to training for teaching staff. A broader application of this hierarchy in the field of speech and language therapy would replace 'student learning outcomes' with 'outcomes for people with communication impairment' or similar. The specific population under consideration would vary depending on the training provided, so it could be all adults admitted to a particular stroke unit following training to nursing staff involved in their care. An alternative could be outcomes for children leaving a range of early years settings if training had been provided to all children's centre staff in a given locality.

A necessary addition to this hierarchy is cost effectiveness. To what extent has the funding required to set up and run the training resulted in measurable savings in terms of short-term issues (reduction in number of referrals to speech and language therapy, for example) and long term (increased economic independence of individuals with communication impairment)?

In order to identify the specific enquiry you have with regard to the evaluation of your training, questions based on Guskey's hierarchy can be used to help focus your thinking. Specifically, to what extent do you want to know what your participants thought of your training programme and how you might improve it in future? Or rather, are you more interested to know about the impact the training will have for clients with communication and feeding/swallowing difficulties? These two extremes cover a range of possible lines of enquiry and very probably you are interested in more than one level of the hierarchy.

The next step in refining your question, therefore, is to identify the range of areas you are interested in, narrow these down to specific queries and then assess the feasibility of finding answers to them. Table 7.1 suggests types of questions for each stage of the hierarchy to help you with refining your questions.

Table 7.1 Levels of evaluation and associated research questions.

Levels of evaluation (adapted from Guskey, 2000)	Nature of enquiry	Possible research questions
Participants' reaction	What did the participants feel about the course?	Did participants enjoy the course? Did participants find the course useful? Did it address participants' needs? Did participants think the course was well-presented and well-organized? How do participants rate their confidence in dealing with individuals with communication impairment following the course compared with before the course?
Participants' learning	To what extent did participants' knowledge, skills, and abilities improve post-training?	Were the objectives of the course met in terms of the aims of the course leaders/commissioners? What new knowledge have course participants acquired? How have the attitudes of the course participants changed following their attendance on the course? What new skills and abilities have course participants acquired?
Organization support and change	How has the organization changed in response to its members/staff attending the training?	Have policies in the organization been altered in light of information given in the training? Is the organization more aware of the importance of communication? Has the organization taken steps to make their environment more communication friendly?
Participants' use of new knowledge and skills	How has participants' behaviour changed in response to the training?	Do participants use the new skills and abilities acquired in the training? In which contexts do participants use these new skills? Are participants using their new skills appropriately and accurately?
Outcomes for individuals with communication impairment	What impact has the training had on individuals with communication impairment?	How do individuals with communication impairment think that their interactions with course participants have changed post training? Have academic, work and/or social outcomes for individuals with communication impairment improved since the course? Have communication skills or opportunities increased in individuals with communication impairment since the course?
Cost effectiveness	Does the course result in economic gains which outweigh the costs of the training?	Are referrals to speech and language therapy reduced from those organizations whose participants attended the training? Are long-term outcomes in terms of economic independence improved for individuals with communication impairment as a result of the course?

Although your specific questions will be particular to your needs and those of whoever has commissioned the evaluation, you may find that you can adapt the suggestions here to suit your requirements. Remember that your questions need to be clearly defined – see Chapter 2 for more detail on this.

These questions are clearly inter-related. An increase in confidence is usually brought about through improved understanding and knowledge. A change in behaviour has to be preceded by a change in skills and increased knowledge or awareness. However, the relationship is not straightforward. Simply knowing what to do does not automatically ensure that what should be done is indeed done.

Nevertheless, if you have decided that you want to focus your question on changes in behaviour, be aware that behaviours can be hard to change and take time and persistence in most cases. As a consequence, evaluating changes in behaviour can be tricky and is inevitably time-consuming. Indeed, a study on the impact of CPD in schools found that most evaluations are restricted to the level of participants' reactions and learning with only a minority evaluating organizational support and change and even fewer considering the impact for the individual child (Goodall, Day, Lindsay, Muijs, & Harris, 2005).

Moreover, while many training programmes are geared up to providing participants with knowledge and skills, many could miss out the crucial element on how to change habits and behaviours. If we are asking individuals to change the way in which they speak to our clients, something which they have done automatically for many years in some cases, then we are asking them to change a behaviour which is very ingrained.

There are, however, possible ways round this tricky issue of centring your question around changes in behaviour. A recent study by Crosskeys and Vance (2011), for example, investigated changes in teacher behaviour through questionnaires completed by their pupils. Specifically, they wanted to know whether pupils had perceived changes in their teachers' behaviours regarding their ability to support children's listening and understanding in the classroom following delivery of a training programme. The training provided to the teachers covered a range of factors of which supporting listening and understanding in the classroom was just one element. However, Crosskeys and Vance focused their attention on this area specifically, refining their question to 'Do pupils perceive any changes in teachers' practice following training?' Focusing their question on one specific area in this way enabled them to identify specific techniques which could answer this question in response to a specific training programme.

Another useful example of questions focusing on changes in behaviour or practice comes from Sorin-Peters, McGilton and Rochon (2010). They took their evaluation to the next level to consider the impact on the individual with communication impairment. Their evaluation was of a training programme for nurses working with individuals with communication impairment in a continuing care setting. Nurses were trained in the use of communication plans, a one-page document giving specific details of an individual's speech, language and communication characteristics and the means through which others can communicate with them, for specific individual clients. A range of measures was used in the evaluation, but in terms of changes for the individual clients, nurses were asked to rate their perception of the usefulness of the communication plans eight weeks after implementation. Whilst this is not a direct measure of the clients' capabilities, this approach is considering the impact of changes made as a result of training to individual clients as perceived by the practitioner.

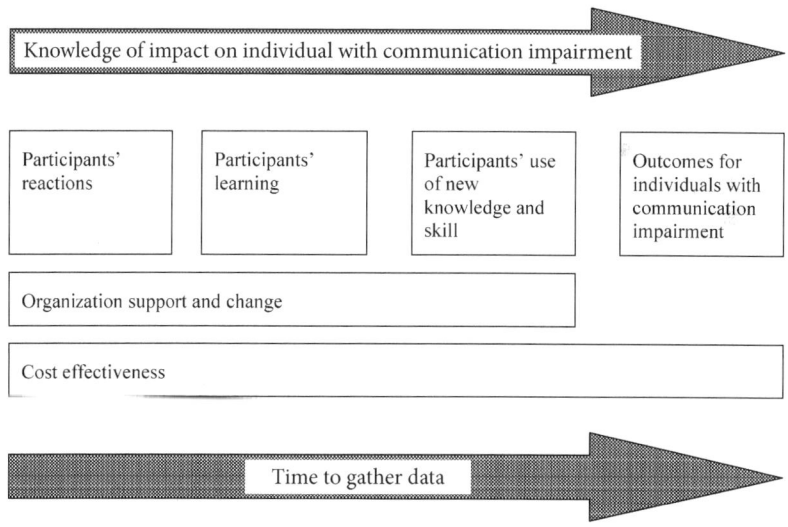

Figure 7.1 Levels of evaluation relative to impact on individuals with communication impairment and time.

To help in narrowing the field for your question, Figure 7.1 illustrates how different levels of enquiry can provide us with varying levels of information in terms of impact on the individual with communication impairment. However, it also shows that, in general, the stronger our knowledge of the impact on the individual, the greater the time investment. The impact of change to organizations will depend on the type of change made. Some changes will have a marked impact – for example, if a setting starts to use symbols as part of its signage thus making the environment more accessible to individuals with certain types of communication impairment. However, other changes which result from training may have a less direct impact, such as changes in policy regarding liaison between one group of professionals and speech and language therapists.

Similarly with cost effectiveness, some changes will have a direct impact on individuals with communication impairment if savings made through the course free up monies that can be used in other ways such as to provide communication aids. In other cases, however, cost savings may be long term and any appreciable benefit for our clients will be negligible.

Both organization changes and cost-effectiveness evaluations can take place in the short term or over a long period of time. In terms of the impact for individuals with communication impairment, however, evaluations are nearly always lengthy as gains in skills made by those trained will take time to show an effect in clients.

The information in Figure 7.1 can help you identify the specific nature of your question and the degree to which it will tell you something about the impact of your training on the individuals whose needs are being targeted. It will also help you to gauge the likely time commitment required to fully answer your query.

So having identified the specific area you want to focus on in your evaluation and refined your question down to one which you think you have the skills, capacity and time to answer, the next step is to identify the most appropriate method to answer it.

What methods will I need to answer my question?

The evaluation of any training programme could effectively be an experimental study – i.e., an investigation measuring the impact of an 'intervention' (in this case a training programme) – on individuals. This requires the investigator to have some knowledge of participants' understanding and behaviours both before and after they are exposed to the 'intervention'.

However, evaluation of training could include either quantitative or qualitative approaches. Your choice of method will be determined by the nature of your question and whether you are interested in larger-scale number data which can be analyzed statistically, or more detailed descriptive data. The approaches are not mutually exclusive and, depending on your research question and the resources available to you, it is feasible to use a combination of both types, allowing for 'triangulation' of your data which adds validity to your findings.

Both qualitative and quantitative methods are valuable in terms of expanding our knowledge base and, in the specific area of evaluating training, understanding the impact of a course. However, the methods will generate different data sets, findings and conclusions so it is important to consider what you want to achieve from your evaluation.

Quantitative approaches

If your aim is to identify broad generalizable findings which can be applied in a range of settings – for example, appraising a large-scale training programme for learning support assistants in a range of schools, in order to understand its potential impact if rolled out to more schools – then quantitative approaches will be most suitable.

For your evaluation to qualify as a true experiment, a control group who is not exposed to the 'intervention' or training should be included and participants should be randomly assigned to either the control or the 'experimental' group. In many clinical situations, this is unlikely to be possible. A 'quasi-experimental' design where a non-equivalent control group is used might be more feasible. This does not require randomization of participants and enables the researcher to use pre-assigned groups. For example, in a pre-school setting or nursing home where only half the staff are able to attend the training (as the other half are on duty), a non-equivalent control group who may be willing to be included in the evaluation is easily available.

In most cases, however, it will not be possible to identify any sort of control group. Where a single group pre-test, post-test design is used, it is referred to as a pre-experimental design. The lack of a control group leads to problems with validity as a range of other influences could be affecting the group and accounting for changes in knowledge, attitudes and behaviour. Indeed, simply the act of being measured for the evaluation could result in unintended impacts. As clinician researchers, there is a need to recognize these limitations and seek to minimize them whilst maintaining a practical and realistic approach to the evaluation.

In an ideal situation, you may be able to use a time-series design where multiple observations are made both pre- and post- training. Crosskeys and Vance (2011) used this approach in their study. Pupils were asked to complete questionnaires on their teachers' use of strategies to promote listening and understanding amongst pupils in the classroom. The questionnaire was administered eight weeks prior to the training and immediately before the training was delivered, in order to assess for the 'Hawthorne' effect, i.e., the effect that might take place by simply engaging in a project regardless of the intervention. The post-training questionnaire could then be used with greater validity to show change as a consequence of the training.

In many situations, however, funding and time limitations plus willingness of course participants could well make this approach impossible. More realistically, you as the clinician researcher will need to consider any other possible influences that could account for any changes post training in your participants. These could be broad ranging and include new curriculum demands for teaching staff, changes to regulations for nursing home care assistants, alternative working arrangements for other professional groups and self-education of parents through use of the internet and other available sources. Whilst knowing about these factors does not allow you to fully account for their impact, it does help to provide a fuller picture and enables you to acknowledge the possible influence that these factors might have had on your participants' response to the training.

Qualitative approaches

Qualitative approaches are useful if you are interested in understanding the specific mechanism of how training others in a particular skill impacts on an identified deficit in individuals with communication impairment. For example, training carers how to support children with profound and multiple learning difficulties with feeding might require observation of those carers using their new techniques in practice. Such observation will provide feedback to the course providers on the effectiveness of their teaching approaches and guidance on how the course could be improved.

You might also want to gain a deeper insight into participants' responses to the training through qualitative approaches which use interviews or focus groups as a means of data collection. Alternatively, ethnographic approaches using observation and video analysis can provide useful ways of understanding the impact of your training in real-life situations and amongst specific groups of participants and clients.

More information on qualitative approaches can be found in Silverman (2009) listed under Further Reading at the end of the chapter. In addition, many of the chapters in this book consider the use of quantitative and qualitative approaches to data collection while Chapter 2 gives a good overview.

Getting into the detail

Once you have decided on which method to use, based on your research questions and the type of information you want to generate, the next steps are to decide on the who, what, when and where of data collection.

Sample

The first decision – who – refers to which individuals are going to form your sample. Where quantitative approaches are used, you are likely to want to include all course participants and indeed, if possible, identify a control group as described above. Where qualitative methods will be employed, you may prefer to use a smaller sample of participants, in which case you must be clear about how these individuals have been selected. You may have specific inclusion and exclusion criteria based on which participants are the 'best fit' for your particular question. Alternatively, more practical considerations might influence your choice, such as which participants work in an environment where video observation is possible. Whatever the rationale behind your inclusion criteria, or indeed if your selection is random, this must be carefully documented.

Data collection

The next major factor relates to data collection. What will you collect? When will you collect it? Where will you collect it? This will vary depending on whether you are using a quantitative or qualitative approach and also depending on the type of research question you are asking. The next section considers the methods of data collection in relation to these issues in more detail; however, in addition to your choice of method, a crucial question will be when to collect the data. Evaluation of training will in many cases require a 'before' and 'after' phase in order to consider the effect of the training on any behaviour, skill or knowledge. There is sometimes a tendency to consider evaluation as simply a post-training activity, but for many research questions linked to evaluation of training you will need to consider when and how to collect data pre-training. Wren (2003), Sorin-Peters et al. (2010) and Crosskeys and Vance (2011) all included pre-training assessments as part of their evaluations.

Related to this factor is the issue of where you will collect the data. Post training is generally easier to collect as you can ask participants to fill in post training evaluations or agree with participants how you will follow up the training with them through observations post course, etc. To collect pre-training data, you will need to ensure you have contact details for all prospective course attendees and liaise with them regarding your method of pre-course data collection. Some types of data are easier to collect than others and you will need to consider this in your planning.

Where the method of data collection involves direct contact with the course participants, for example through interviews or observations, comparing pre- and post-training data is most reliable when the person collecting the post-training data is blinded. In other words, the observer/interviewer is unaware of the status or level of knowledge and skill that the individual had prior to the course or, indeed, during the course and therefore is less biased in their collection of this data. Wherever possible, it is advisable to identify an individual who has not been involved in pre-training data collection or in the running of the course to carry out the post-test data collection. An approach using blinding in course evaluations is described in Crosskeys and Vance (2011).

Having established that your basic research methodology is that of an experiment, the next issue to consider is what type of data collection to use. Table 7.2 shows the most suitable methods of data collection for use in evaluating training in relation to the types of question you might ask. Different levels of evaluation are considered under the two broad groupings of quantitative and qualitative approaches

Table 7.2 Methods of data collection related to levels of evaluation.

Level of evaluation Method of data collection		Participants' reactions	Participants' learning	Organization change and support	Participants' use of new knowledge and skills	Outcomes for individuals with communication impairment	Cost effectiveness
Quantitative methods	Questionnaires to participants	X	X	X	X		
	Documentary evidence			X		X	X
	Assessment of individuals with communication impairment				X	X	
Qualitative methods	Interviews of participants	X	X	X	X		
	Interviews of individuals with communication impairment				X	X	
	Documentary evidence			X		X	X
	Reflective logs/journals		X		X		
	Observations				X	X	
	Focus groups of participants	X	X	X	X		
	Focus groups of individuals with communication impairment					X	
	Role play/task simulation				X		
	Case study	X	X	X	X	X	X

Questionnaires

In terms of quantitative approaches, questionnaires post training are a commonly used way of gaining feedback on a course. When a questionnaire is used pre- and post-training, it can be used to provide information relating to participants' learning, organization change and support and their use of new knowledge and skills. Sorin-Peters et al. (2010) and Crosskeys and Vance (2011) both used questionnaires, delivered both pre- and post-training, to evaluate their courses. The questionnaires were used to evaluate participant learning, use of new knowledge and skills and outcomes for individuals with communication impairment.

Three main types of question can be used depending on the kind of information you want to extract. Closed questions are useful for factual information and for when you want to limit the possible responses. This is useful if your aim is to count responses and provide percentage style data in terms of participants' response to your training. You can also use some open-ended questions which can be helpful in providing quotes and detail to support your numerical data in reports and feedback. Avoid using many open-ended questions, however, as analyzing these requires the use of qualitative techniques and can be time-consuming.

Rating scales

A third style of question – rating scales – can be particularly useful in gaining information about individuals' attitudes to the training and their perception of their own confidence and learning. A typical rating scale question will start with a statement and the respondent is asked to indicate to what extent they agree with that statement. These scales can be easily converted to numerical data, making analysis more straightforward. Scales such as these were used by Wren (1999) to compare teachers' self-rating of their confidence and knowledge.

Bear in mind the possible disadvantages of using such scales, however. For example, can you be sure that respondents have a consistent internal rating scale when they respond pre- and post-training? For more information on questionnaire design and attitude measurement, see Oppenheim (2000), listed under Further Reading.

Documentary evidence

Documentary evidence can consist of a range of material from minutes of meetings to performance tables, inspection reports and planning documents.

The primary purpose of these documents will be related to operational issues rather than for the evaluation of a training programme but they can provide a useful source of evidence for the clinician researcher. Specifically, if the researcher clinician is interested in knowing about organization change and support pre- and post-training, then the minutes of meetings, policies and planning documents can be invaluable. Performance tables such as schools' SATs can provide data on change in performance over time, allowing a comparison of performance pre- and post-training. Given that the nature of documentary evidence could be either numerical or text data, it is included under both quantitative and qualitative methods.

Cost effectiveness can also be measured using existing data sets. Statistical data on numbers of referrals and time spent on SLT caseloads for particular client groups, for example, can be explored using NHS datasets. Make sure you are clear about your expectations regarding change post training, however. Was the aim of your training to increase referrals, as participants were made more aware of the contribution of SLT for their clients, or was it designed to reduce referrals, on the basis that participants would be better equipped to deal with many of the problems themselves?

As described above, documentary evidence can also be used to provide qualitative data. Specifically, it can be used to provide information relative to organizational change, impacts on the individual clients and cost effectiveness. The detail provided in these documents, when analyzed using qualitative techniques, can provide a useful adjunct to the quantitative evaluation.

Client assessments

Direct assessment of individuals with communication impairment can shed light on changes at this level post training. Formal assessments are best at providing quantitative data though some informal assessments can be quantified. Collation of results for several clients will provide a more robust evaluation of the impact of the training than reporting on one or two individuals.

An example of when you might want to collect data relating to a client's impairment might be when a child is receiving indirect intervention from a speech and language therapist and the SLT wants to assess the impact of the input from a learning support assistant following training in the child's specific area of need.

It is essential that baseline data is obtained for each of the clients assessed prior to the training. It is also important to consider the length of time it might take course participants to implement new skills and techniques into their everyday practice. As a consequence, measuring change in individual clients should take place some time after the training has completed in order to allow time for the participant to make changes and time for those changes to take effect. Indeed, both Sorin-Peters et al. (2010) and Crosskeys and Vance (2011) waited until eight weeks post training to collect their post-training evaluation data.

Interviews and focus groups

In terms of the qualitative approaches listed in Table 7.2, interviews and focus groups with either participants or clients can be useful ways to get more information than is possible with a questionnaire. Responses could be recorded, allowing for later transcription; this can be time-consuming so make sure you allow enough time and funding for this in your plans.

Logs and journal

Reflective logs and journals are alternatives and will provide you with a ready source of written reports from course participants, thus avoiding the need for transcription. Participants could be asked to record their work practices in their log, allowing you as the researcher to identify changes to their practice over time.

Observation

The disadvantages of interviews, focus groups and reflective logs and journals, however, are that they all rely on self-report. An alternative would be to observe the course participants in their work or home setting both pre- and post-training in order to observe possible changes to their behaviours. This approach can be costly in terms of time, requiring an individual to visit each participant and spend time observing them. It is possible to film participants or, indeed, ask participants to record themselves, though there is the issue with both live and recorded observations that typical practice is altered by the presence of an observer or recording equipment.

Role play and task simulation

Using role play or task simulation can often produce a negative response in participants who dislike this learning style. However, as a means to investigate skills and behaviours they can be useful tools. Whilst they do not provide information on whether the participants actually use their new skills in everyday activities, they do at least provide evidence regarding participants' ability to use newly-acquired skills.

In the evaluation of the training provided to teaching staff described in Wren (2003), task simulations were used in the form of scenarios. Each scenario described a particular pupil with a type of communication impairment and a context for the classroom, such as teaching a specific technique in maths. The teachers were asked questions regarding the child's potential difficulties in this situation and also how they could help facilitate the child's learning in that lesson. The scenarios were completed pre- and post-training, thus allowing the researcher to understand the impact that the training had made on teachers' ability to use their new knowledge without the need to carry out lengthy in-class observations.

Case studies

A case study approach allows the clinician researcher to investigate one, or at most a few, participants in detail. In this situation, the researcher can investigate a range of questions across one or two participants rather than a single question across a range of participants. This approach has the advantage of being able to consider the impact of a particular training course across a range of parameters. It can be used to evaluate performance in terms of a participant's learning, organization change and support, participant's use of their new knowledge and skills, impact on that participant's clients and subsequent cost effectiveness.

The disadvantage of this approach, however, is the fact that a single case study could involve an atypical participant who has responded to the training in a way which is categorically different to other participants on the course. This could give you unusually positive or negative findings – but without information on other participants there is no way of knowing which. A case series design, where a series of case studies are carried out, can be a useful way to increase the validity and reliability of this approach.

In summary, there are no ideal methods of data collection in terms of evaluating course outcomes. The most sensible approach is, first, to consider what type of information you need (quantitative or qualitative) in relation to your research question. This will help you identify the most appropriate method. Combined methods, however, provide an opportunity to triangulate your information which will add validity to your findings. Second, consider the resources available to you and limitations and constraints imposed. As a clinician researcher, your time and funding for these endeavours are likely to be more restricted than those operating in a pure research environment such as a university academic department and therefore what is possible is likely to be more limited. Nevertheless, being aware of the pitfalls of each approach means you will be best placed to minimize them as far as is possible while acknowledging the unavoidable limitations in any subsequent report.

Ethical considerations

In order to comply with ethics regulations, ensure that any data you do collect is anonymized and that access to this data is restricted to those working on the evaluation. Be mindful as well when designing questionnaires and other methods of data collection that all questions or enquiries that are included can be justified in terms of your research questions and that no unnecessary personal information is requested. This is particularly important as we consider how you will store and manage your data.

Managing the data

As you collect data for your evaluation, you will need to ensure that you have systematic ways of storing and collating it. This will vary depending on the nature of the data but of vital importance is ensuring that your data is collated in such a way that it can be accessed easily when required and can be analyzed reliably. You may be able to access some administrative help to assist you in this process but you will need to decide and set up the process in the first place.

If you are collecting quantitative data, ensure you have a means to identify which has been collected or retrieved and which you are still waiting for. Categorize the types of data you will be collecting so that as documents or questionnaires arrive through the post, you are able to quickly file them ready for when you need to access them for analysis.

With regards to qualitative data, consider how the data would be best organized. If you are carrying out two or three single case studies or observations, you might want to write a checklist for each participant to keep track of which data you have obtained and which still needs to be sought. It could suit your needs to file all data according to each participant or according to the type of data depending on your particular investigation.

Analysis

This stage is the crucial one where all your hard work in collecting pre-training data, carrying out the training itself and ensuring that post-test data is collected comes together to provide an answer to your original question.

The type of analysis will again depend on the nature of your research question and the type of data you have collected. The level of analysis will also vary according to the level of skill and experience you have and the amount of access you have to others who can help you.

With regard to quantitative data, a range of statistical techniques can be used to answer your question. In terms of questionnaires, frequency counts or percentages can be used to describe how many participants responded to each option for closed questions (for example, girl/boy, impaired/typical). Other descriptive statistics such as means, standard deviations and ranges can be calculated for continuous data (for example, age, test scores). Depending upon your research design, a range of statistical analyses can be used to calculate the degree of change between pre- and post-training means, including t-tests, ANOVA and chi-squared statistics. These will provide information on the strength of evidence in your data and, in some instances, subsequent analyses can be used to describe the direction. For more information on these and other similar statistical techniques, see Hinton (2004) listed in Further Reading.

Where open questions have been included in the questionnaire, these can provide useful quotes to back up your numerical findings, making a subsequent report a more enjoyable and illuminating read.

Scaled questions can also be analyzed in this way when points along the scale are ascribed numerical value. For example, if the answer, 'agree strongly' was given the value of 1 and 'disagree strongly' given 5, scores for these responses before and after training could be compared for all participants. Alternatively, the degree of change pre- and post-training could be quantified.

Assessment of individuals with communication impairment can be analyzed using quantitative approaches where the data provided is either already numerical or can be converted to numerical data (for example, checklists where scores for number of items achieved are used or informal assessments where clinical judgement is used to give the client a score).

Documentary evidence can be analyzed using either statistical methods or qualitative approaches depending on the type of data in the document. Where numerical data are available, some statistical analyses may already have been performed for you (for example SATs data).

With text data, qualitative approaches will need to be used. One possible approach is to use thematic analysis in which emergent themes are identified in the data set. In order to do this, the researcher needs to be very familiar with their data and in many cases will need to code their data prior to analysis. In other words, they need to read through the data and note particular emergent themes and code each theme. This can be a time-consuming process, adding extra weight to the message regarding not to collect too much data! As highlighted earlier in the section 'Refining your question', be clear what your specific question is and try to collect and analyze data which brings you closer to answering that specific query.

Notes and transcriptions from interviews, observations, focus groups, case studies and journal/logs can all be analyzed using a thematic approach. The key issue in the analysis of qualitative data pre- and post-training will be the degree to which themes can be identified which show change following participation in a specific training activity.

Role play and simulation techniques can allow for a more targeted approach to analyzing qualitative data as the amount of data collected may be reduced. The activities can also be constructed to ensure that only the data required is collected. Analysis of this sort of data will be a more straightforward comparison of responses pre- and post-training and could be useful when wanting to establish whether a participant has acquired skills that he or she did not previously possess.

It is important to remember at this stage what other possible influences could have exerted an effect on your sample. This is particularly important in the cases where no control group has been recruited and where the effects of the training might take some time to show. It could be very difficult or even impossible to quantify the relative contribution that other influences may have had on the sample but acknowledging them is still important. Where individual data are reported, as in case studies of course participants or clients with communication impairment, it is important to acknowledge the difficulty with applying findings universally and the possibility that the case used is unique rather than typical.

Conclusions

So in terms of providing training – does it make a difference? Well quite possibly yes – but don't take it for granted. Evaluating training is important but make sure you are clear you know why you want to evaluate it and for what outcome. Be clear about what you are trying to achieve through the training and therefore what questions need to be asked. And be sure to at least consider possible ways of measuring the impact of the training, not just the perception of the participants. Increased confidence and knowledge is of less value than change to practice as a consequence of advances in these areas. And finally, be realistic about what you can achieve. We all operate within time and funding constraints – consider what yours are and therefore what is feasible to measure in the time and space you have available. Better a small quality evaluation than a large-scale enquiry which is never completed.

Summary

This chapter provides guidance on the stages to go through in order to effectively answer the chapter title question. The first step is to identify what sort of difference you are hoping for. Once you are clear about that – and it is a view that is shared with participants on any training and funders, then it is possible to refine your question to one that can be answered. This involves considering both theoretical and practical issues in order to come up with a question which is feasible and which fits with your original enquiry.

With a clearly-defined question in mind, the sample, type of methodology and most suitable method of data collection can be identified; bearing in mind the crucial factor of collecting pre- as well as post-course data.

With a systematic method of data collation in place, subsequent analysis can take place in a timely and organized fashion. Findings can then be considered in light of what is already known in the field and the context in which the training is being carried out. The final step of writing up and disseminating results is essential, though your intended audience will vary depending on the initial purpose of your evaluation. If funders need a formal report on the evaluation then you may be able to provide a summary version for participants and your employer. If the purpose of the evaluation was for your own benefit to appraise the value of a specific programme, then you may be satisfied with a simple collation of your findings. However, it would be a shame for the effort you will undoubtedly have put into the evaluation to be limited in this way. Consider writing a brief report or presentation which you can use with your employers or other potential funders or, indeed, future participants. It is important for the profession that as many people as possible know about the benefits or limitations of any training we deliver so that they can identify which types of CPD have most value in their fields. So having done all that work, don't keep it to yourself, share it and tell others.

The process of evaluating training in a way which provides reliable and meaningful data is not easy and not as straightforward as carrying out a simple post-course evaluation form. However, it is essential in order to inform best practice in our profession and for our clients. It can be costly in terms of time and effort but the benefits of knowing that you have done a good job, that you have had an effect, that you have indeed made a difference, should not be underestimated.

References

Crosskeys, E. & Vance, M. (2011) Training teachers to support pupils' listening in class: An evaluation using pupil questionnaires. *Child Language Teaching and Therapy* **27:2,** 165–182.

Goodall, J., Day, C., Lindsay, G., Muijs, D., & Harris, A. (2005) *Evaluating the Impact of Continuing Professional Development (CPD).* (No. RR659). Nottingham: DFES.

Guskey, T. R. (2000) *Evaluating Professional Development.* Thousand Oaks, California: Corwin Press.

Oldroyd, D. & Hall, V. (1991) *Managing Staff Development: A Handbook for Secondary Schools.* London: Chapman Hall.

Sorin-Peters, R., McGilton, K. S., & Rochon, E. (2010) The development and evaluation of a training programme for nurses working with persons with communication disorders in a complex continuing care facility. *Aphasiology* **24:12,** 1511–1536.

Wren, Y. (2003) Using scenarios to evaluate a professional development programme for teaching staff. *Child Language Teaching and Therapy* **19:2,** 115–134.

Wren, Y. (1999) An Evaluation of a Professional Development Programme for Teaching Staff. Unpublished Masters thesis.

Further reading

Hinton, P. (2004) *Statistics Explained: A Guide for Social Science Students*. Hove: Routledge.

Oppenheim, A. N. (2000) *Questionnaire Design, Interviewing and Attitude Measurement*. London: Continuum.

Silverman, D. (2009) *Doing Qualitative Research* (2nd edition). London: Sage.

8 How many clients do I have that...? Gathering data from existing sources

Jan Broomfield

> ### Learning outcomes
>
> By the end of this chapter, you will be able to:
>
> - Identify your individual or your service's caseload
> - Work out how many clients face a particular issue
> - Think about the outcomes of the service being provided

Introduction

In this chapter, I will guide busy working clinicians and service managers on how to gather data in their own clinical contexts, which can inform service planning, as well as funding and commissioning bodies and the research agenda. Much of this information can be gathered from existing records, and if this is done systematically it ensures that the findings are useful – and can be repeated in subsequent years so that comparisons can be made over time.

What are the clinical issues or challenges?

Service managers are frequently asked about the recipients of their service, their numbers, and their epidemiological distribution (for example, what they 'look' like, how old they are, how many new assessments are seen, etc.) or their clinical presentations. How readily are you able to provide the answers to these questions?

It is possible, with a little organization, to gather this information and store it in an accessible format. This is enhanced by the increased access to computerized patient systems, which can collect specific information to serve your purpose. Some questions can be answered by looking back at case notes, computerized records and tallies such as 'how many new referrals were received in a specific time frame?' Others, such as 'how effective is the service you offer?', may require planning and organization to enable future collection of relevant data.

This chapter will pose potential questions that you might wish to ask, and discuss how you might answer them. Three broad questions are identified at this stage, and will be used to illustrate the process of data gathering and analysis throughout the chapter:

1. *How many clients does your service see?* This is the sort of question that is likely to be asked by those who fund your services. It is particularly helpful to be able to answer this when predicting how many clients you expect to be seen in the coming year; information that may be required when you are negotiating contracts or funding for on-going services.

2. *How many clients are identified at initial contact as requiring further input from your service?* This question may come from a central or local multi-agency funding body, so that they can plan for future potential needs, considering their own funding budgets.

3. *How successful is the service you offer?* This question relates to outcomes and can be tailored to your specific service, looking at different clinical populations separately.

What do we already know about the issue?

You need to know what is already available regarding the question you are trying to answer, because this helps to put your service into a national context, and may enable you to make comparisons with what the evidence base indicates.

For question 1, 'How many clients does your service see?', you could look at national published data, perhaps available from your professional body, and compare your service with others of similar population size and socio-economic distribution. There may be papers published in peer-reviewed journals which discuss caseload size and epidemiological information, which would provide a baseline for comparison.

For question 2, 'How many clients are identified at initial contact as requiring further input from your service?', you could look again at peer-reviewed papers to identify typical proportions of referrals who then require further intervention.

For question 3, 'How successful is the service you offer?', you would need to identify literature that has been published about clinical outcomes and service discharges, for a comparable clinical population, which again would provide a baseline.

Furthermore, these publications could guide you in determining the methods and measures to use; this is discussed later in this chapter.

Literature searching

When searching a database for relevant literature, it is essential that you identify relevant 'search terms' to ensure that you find a selection of papers which are specific to your question, without identifying too many to be helpful. This means that your question must be specific and precise. You can then identify the key words in your question – these will form the terms you use for your literature search.

Your question can be formulated to help with your search, using the mnemonic PICO (Richardson et al., 1995). Using this approach, '**P**' refers to problem or patient, i.e., the problem or patient group you are interested in. You then enter the clinical condition as your 'P' search term. For example, you could identify school-aged children with language difficulty, adults with learning difficulties or teachers with dysphonia. It could be beneficial to seek literature specifying the incidence and/or prevalence of your particular clinical presentation; you will then be able to make evidence-based predictions about the anticipated referral rate, and compare your caseload size with this.

The 'I' in PICO represents intervention or exposure: what is being done to the client or what possible exposure is of interest. Specify the particular intervention, if appropriate, or just state 'therapy' or 'intervention' if you wish to look for a broad range of evidence. '**C**' stands for comparison: you might wish to look for articles that consider an alternate intervention or, indeed, no intervention. If you are considering changing the intervention approach that you use with your specified client group, then search for the new intervention in the 'I' element, and your current intervention in 'C'. You will then be able to compare the effects of each and make an evidence-informed decision.

The 'O' refers to outcome, i.e., what is the desired outcome of your intervention. For example, you may specify 'improved language', 'return to work' or 'independence' for each of the examples above.

So, your resulting search terms for each of the PICO elements from these examples could be:

(a) Children, language difficulties, narrative therapy, improved language

(b) Adults, learning difficulties, social skills intervention, independence

(c) Adults, dysphonia, intervention, return to work

It is also worth looking at the evidence that has been produced by your professional body. For example, the Royal College of Speech and Language Therapists (RCSLT) has recently produced and commissioned a range of evidence-based documents, including:

- The Commissioning Resource Manual (RCSLT, 2009), a synthesis of the best available research for a range of clinical areas, including learning disabilities, speech and language impairment and voice.

- The Matrix Report (RCSLT, 2010), an analysis of the cost benefits of specific areas of speech and language therapy (SLT), specifically Specific Language Impairment, autism and stroke.

- A range of Position Papers and Policy Statements, each of which provides a summary of the best evidence, together with statements recommending the optimum management, for a range of specific clinical conditions.

Other professional organizations often make Position Statements and Evidence Summaries available on their website. Examples of these include The American Speech Hearing Association (ASHA), which has a comprehensive website, and SpeechBITE (University of Sydney and Speech Pathology Australia), which is a database providing open access to a catalogue of Best Interventions and Treatment Efficacy across a scope of SLT practice (see Resources section at the end of the chapter).

Even if these documents and websites do not provide the specific answer to your evidence search, they will have helpful background information as well as a wide relevant reference list. It may be that these references provide you with an initial start point for your reading.

Support networks

There is a wide range of sources of support for clinicians and service managers wishing to undertake studies of their population. These include:

- Clinical forums which may be online, through professional bodies or through local universities; each encourages discussion about specific issues and sharing of experiences.

- Special Interest Groups (SIGs) or Clinical Excellence Networks, which often focus on specific client groups; across the UK, the RCSLT has established a network of these groups, and as part of the affiliation to the professional body asks that they engage in evidence-based practice or research activities.

- Colleagues in academia or research, who are always available and open to discuss mechanisms by which they can support local projects, particularly where this may in turn support student placements, student projects or academic research.

- Consultant SLT and specialist clinical advisors and their respective professional networks, who again are experts in a particular clinical field; in addition, they have often engaged in research or service evaluation.

- Local authorities or councils, who often collect and analyze data about their total populations; for example, national census data are analyzed on a local level to enable population service planning such as education, transport and employment issues. These sources can provide information such as total population, ethnic typography, socio-economic make-up and other demographic detail. Knowing the make-up of the local population helps to place a clinical population in context and, in turn, can assist service planning.

- Local Health Research Networks (comprehensive local research networks) are established across the UK, and use a range of professionals including experienced researchers, statisticians and health economists, specifically to help and support local research within health services.

Refining the question

Typically, the type of question you'll ask of your caseload, whether all or part, will originate from either a clinical or contractual query. This could be requested by your team, manager, funder, commissioner or a service user. It is essential that you identify the level of detail that is required in order that your findings are fit for purpose. Better to spend time at the start, making sure you have asked the right question, than get to the end and realize that your report does not fulfil the required objective or omits an essential piece of information.

The question you are asked, and the resulting research question that you need to answer, is often in the form of 'how many' or 'what type', and could also have a financial element associated with it. It is important that you refine your question to make it as specific as possible to your needs, so that you identify exactly what you want to know. You should avoid asking general questions, or your literature search and your data collection will be too broad and become unmanageable; your resulting findings will not be detailed enough to meet your needs. Being clear about the purpose of your investigation, and the intended audience, can help to guide you in identifying the particular issue in question.

Considerations when refining your question include:

- Specifying a particular clinical population – for example, if your service provides for all adults with acquired disorders, you might wish to find information relating only to progressive neurological conditions.

- Identifying a particular referral source or sector – for example, if you are responding to a question from a social care organization, it might not be helpful to tell them about health care referrals.

- Identifying a particular age group – for example, if your question comes from the school sector, they probably don't wish to know about neonates.

- Identifying a particular location – for example, if your service covers a broad area, you might need to restrict your search to just one borough.

- Determining a time frame for your data collection – perhaps you want to consider the previous year or three years, or the coming year. This not only helps you in defining the parameters of your data collection, but will guide your literature search. It may be that the last census is within your timeframe, in which case this could be a very useful source of population data.

■ Deciding the outcomes that you wish to consider – it might be that you want to report quantitative results, for example from standardized assessments, reporting impairment levels. Or you might prefer a more functional outcome, such as wellbeing or quality of life measures. You will need to decide which measures you intend to use; again, literature searching could guide you in deciding the most appropriate and effective outcome measure for your client group and your individual needs.

The three questions stated above could be refined as follows:

For question1, 'How many clients does your service see?', you could specify the clinical population, the age range and the time scale you wish to look at. For example, how many school-aged children with language difficulties, adults aged 19 to 65 with learning difficulties, or teachers with dysphonia? You might wish to look at the last year, the last three years, or the coming year.

For question 2, 'How many clients are identified at initial contact as requiring further input from your service?', you could again specify the clinical population, age range and time scale. In addition, you might wish to identify the clinical criteria used by your service to decide that a newly-assessed individual requires further intervention. For example, with children you could consider standardized scores on a particular assessment; for adults with learning difficulties you could identify a particular profile on a functional communication assessment; for teachers with dysphonia you might wish to consider elements of lifestyle which could impact on presentation.

For question 3, 'How successful is the service you offer?', as well as identifying the above issues, you could identify the intervention approach used if this is the same for all those in your chosen client group, as well as the outcomes that you wish to measure. For a group of school-aged children with language difficulties, you might provide narrative therapy and wish to measure improved language or educational attainment. For adults with learning difficulties, you could provide a social skills intervention and measure improvements to independence. For teachers with dysphonia, you might provide a range of interventions then measure return to work as an outcome for the whole client group.

What methods will I need to answer my question?

There are two main methods of gathering data relating to the nature of your caseload and the issues discussed above – retrospective and prospective methods.

Retrospective data collection

Retrospective data collection involves looking back at information you already have in your possession. This could be a matter of running a general count, for example, how many clients received initial assessment, the typical data that a service manager will report on a regular basis, to a breakdown of 'epidemiology', which refers to the detail about your population. The latter could be about such things as age, gender, ethnicity and socio-economic status, and the clinical information such as referral source, presenting condition, severity. This information could already be entered into a pre-existing electronic data storage system from which a summary report can be run, or perhaps require a trawl through client files, seeking specific information.

Once you have decided on the type of information you require, set up a table or a database so that you can record your findings and keep track of where you are up to. It is advisable to keep this data anonymously, but it's worthwhile keeping a separate file, stored safely, which matches the client to the table or database you have developed, in case you wish to add additional information at a later date. A simple table would look like the example shown in Table 8.1. (N.B. Pre-determine the categories you will use, and the criteria for the severity ratings, so that your input is consistent.)

Table 8.1: Sample epidemiological and clinical data collection table.

Client number	Age	Gender	Ethnicity	Referral Source	Presenting Condition	Severity
1	5;6	M	English	School	Language impairment	Moderate
2	7;2	M	English	Parent	Speech disorder	Moderate
3	11;1	F	Pakistani Heritage	School	Language impairment	Moderate
4	3;2	M	Polish	Health Visitor	Language impairment	Severe
etc						

Once the data set is complete, you can then conduct analyses to obtain summaries of the information collected. This will be discussed later in the chapter in the analysis section.

This method of data collection would be appropriate to answer questions about the number of clients seen in a set time period and, subject to the information being available in the records, the epidemiological 'population' information such as age, gender, referral source and presenting condition. It could also be able to identify the level of expertise required by the client following initial assessment. However, that data may not always be apparent in the case notes, in which case it will be necessary to collect the information with new clients. This leads us on to prospective data collection.

Prospective data collection

Here the information required is less typical or less easily retrieved, or information that you have not consistently collected in the past; it will therefore be appropriate to collect the data at forthcoming client appointments.

What is required is a systematic collection of data. It is therefore helpful to adapt your case records, such as case history form, so that the data that you require will be systematically collected. Perhaps you wish to know specific details about the working environments of your dysphonic clients; this might not currently be recorded in the same place in case notes by the assessing clinicians – by adding specific questions to your case history form, or devising a brief questionnaire to be completed by each clinician or client, you can ensure that this information is easily retrievable from client records. If you then set up a database or table with a column for each question and a code or set of criteria for the possible responses, such as in Table 8.1 above, this information can be collected systematically; perhaps it is recorded at the same time as other data is input into a client reporting system, or new assessment files are kept in a particular place until the end of the week, when you systematically work through them to transfer the appropriate data onto your database.

This method of data collection would be appropriate to answer questions relating to information that has not been systematically collected in the past, for example the severity of the presenting condition based on a single, agreed, set of criteria, or outcomes relating not only to the specific intervention undertaken, but in relation to increasing independence or returning to work.

Getting into the detail

What's the question you have been set or have set yourself? Discuss it in detail with colleagues to ensure that you have identified the types of data that you need to collect, how you are going to collect the data, and how you will record what you collect. It is worth specifying criteria for the less clear-cut measures you might record; for example, age is relatively straightforward, but will you record years and months or do you want to include days too? For measures such as outcome or severity, you must identify how you will record these before you start, so that you consistently use the descriptors or scoring system or outcome measures that you establish throughout the time of your data collection. That information is then available to you when you analyze and write up your findings and when you look back in years to come. This clarity is particularly important when more than one person is involved in the data collection or data recording, so that you can be sure that the whole team is consistent and the data are reliable.

You need a protocol which everyone can refer to. This document will describe each step in detail, and includes all the specifications for inclusion criteria, categories of client, age specifications, the measurements that you are using, the outcomes that you have agreed, and any other issue which defines and describes the process you are following and the data that you are collecting. The protocol should be as detailed as possible, so that anyone can read it and know exactly what you are doing. It means that you have sufficient detail to make your study replicable by someone else without them needing to ask you for any information. It also means that you can ensure that you and anyone else involved in the study can refer to the document and be certain that the approach is consistent. It also forms the basis for the introduction and methods sections when you decide to write up your findings for publication.

However, that doesn't mean that you should ask every question you can think of, and collect every response from your existing records or future contacts; not only will you be overburdened with findings, but you will struggle to sift through and identify the responses to the specific issue in question. So, take the time to ensure you are collecting the appropriate amount and level of information from whichever source you use.

Sampling

The purpose of your study is to use the information you gather from a selected sample of individuals to make inferences about the wider population. It may be that you gather data from the next 100 clients seen by your service who fit your criteria, or every suitable referral received over the coming year. However, you will use the findings from this sample to suggest that you would obtain similar results from clients fulfilling the same criteria in the future.

A sample is a selected group from the population of interest. Your sample should be small enough to be manageable, but large enough to be able to make inferences and generalizations of your results to the wider population. The size and nature of your sample will be determined by the question you are striving to answer, your specific inclusion and exclusion criteria, and the numbers you are aiming to achieve.

Gathering data about the whole of your referred population over a set time frame requires no particular selection, but instead needs very clear identification of the questions you'll ask, and investigations you'll undertake, in order to obtain the data you require. But again, you will wish to make inferences about future referrals, so your studied population becomes your sample, and you will generalize your results to future referrals.

Determining sample size

Determining sample size can be a difficult decision. If your sample size is too large, the study will take a long time to complete and will be costly in terms of time and resources. If your sample size is too small, it will be harder to obtain a conclusive answer and to generalize your findings to the wider population.

In qualitative data collection, you can set your study size to suit your question, considering how many of your chosen clients will be available within a manageable time scale. You will need to explain why you have chosen the sample size, and explain what strategies you can put in place if you need to include more clients.

In quantitative data collection, the mechanism for determining how many clients you will include in your sample is more complex. It involves making a power calculation, which estimates how big your sample size should be to be sure that your findings are reliable and generalizable to other clients with the same presentation, or meeting the same criteria. Sample size calculators are available on the internet, but they can be confusing; the best advice is to seek out an experienced researcher or a statistician, perhaps from any of the support networks mentioned earlier.

Data collection and recording

When establishing the nature of the data you wish to collect, consider discussing the detail with your team, your funders and any others who will receive your research report at the end of the study. This will help to ensure that you identify all the elements that you need to include, but avoid collecting data that you will not use.

Confidentiality and anonymity

It is essential that your data collection records remain confidential and are stored securely, for example, in password-protected PC files or in locked filing cabinets. None of these records should contain patient identifiable information, so anonymity must be maintained. However, it is advisable to set up a system whereby you can return to the original file or client in case you require additional information. In this case, each client can be given a pseudonym, with a separate, securely-stored record matching each client with their given pseudonym, so that individuals can be traced if required. This process is known as pseudonymity. For example, if you have few cases in your sample, you could label them alphabetically or, with larger numbers, use figures, for example, 0001 to 1000.

Data collection will now be exemplified using the three question examples posed at the beginning of the chapter.

Question 1: How many clients does your service see?

Much of the data required will be taken retrospectively from your clinical and electronic records; so, once you have established the types of information you need, and set up your recording method, you can go back through clinical records to fill in the detail (retrospective). If you then find gaps in the data you have, you could complete the data collection by finding the answers from subsequent cases seen (prospective). It is advisable to draw up a record sheet onto which your findings can be recorded, whether on paper, on Excel or Access, or some other database. This will ensure that you keep track of where you are up to, as well as form the basis of your later reports. The record sheet should contain all the parameters you wish to measure. Table 8.2 shows an example of measurement of nature of presenting difficulty and severity, relating to children with language difficulties.

Table 8.2: Sample Data Collection Record for Q1 - How many school-aged children with language difficulties have you assessed?

Presentation and severity	Receptive and Expressive	Expressive only	Total
Mild	100	50	150
Moderate	250	75	325
Severe	150	75	225
Total	500	200	700

If you wish to look at severity of presentation, as in Table 8.2, the parameters of each category must be agreed beforehand and specified in your protocol as detailed previously. There are numerous ways of reporting severity and you need to determine which is most appropriate for your needs and your caseload.

For children, you might have undertaken standardized assessments, where you know how other children have performed and can compare each child with others of the same age. If so, you could use any one or any combination of reporting measures, such as raw score, percentile ranking, or age equivalent. Raw scores relate to the actual performance on an assessment, for example the child achieved 7/10 correct responses. Percentile scores show where the individual sits within a normal distribution curve, identifying the percentage of people scoring lower than they have, therefore comparing the individual's score with the population. Age equivalent specifies the equivalent age of functioning of the individual in question, so a 4-year-old could be functioning as a 3-year-old, for example.

Or you could convert these to a more functional scale, by using, for example, the Therapy Outcome Measures [TOMS] (Enderby, John, & Petheram, 2006). This is a tool that enables you to classify individuals according to their impairment, activity/disability, participation and wellbeing, using any or all of the 11 point scales in a systematic way. This type of measurement fits neatly with the World Health Organisation's International Classification of Functioning, Disability and Health (ICF), a framework for consideration of the impact of communication impairment using a holistic approach. For more information on the use of the ICF, see Threats (2006).

For adult populations, you could measure severity by the functional impact that the presenting condition has on the individual's quality of life, as reported by themselves and/or their family. Chapter 6 provides more information on quality of life measures and how to consider a more holistic approach in research.

For further detail on the impact of communication impairment on activity and participation in children, McLeod and Threats (2008) discuss the children and youth version of the ICF and how it applies to a range of assessment and intervention approaches in children with speech disorder.

When considering any of these differing presentations in severity, specify your classification system and criteria in your protocol, in order that the decision-making by others involved is equitable.

Question 2: How many clients are identified at initial assessment as requiring further input from your service?

For this issue, as well as recording whether the intervention is required, it might be appropriate to report according to referral source or residential setting. For example, if your report will be used to inform decisions about your funding sources or payment by results tariffs, it will be important to have information about who has requested assessment of the client. Table 8.3 shows an example of this for our second hypothetical population, adults with learning disabilities.

Table 8.3: Sample Data Collection Record for Q2 - How many adults with learning disabilities require social skills intervention?

Assessment outcome and residential setting	Social skills intervention not required / appropriate	Social skills intervention required	Total
Own home	50	150	200
Social care provision	100	100	200
Health care provision	150	50	200
Total	300	300	600

It is essential to identify exactly what information you wish to report on, and what you don't need. Specifying these issues before you begin to analyze (retrospective) or collect (prospective) data will ensure you find all you need in one go, rather than needing to return and look for a particular aspect at a later date. Better to spend time getting it right first time than needing to revisit your caseload on several occasions.

Question 3: How successful is the service you offer?

There are many ways of measuring outcomes. Your service might have employed a particular framework from the published literature, the evidence base for which is growing. Or you might have adopted a client reporting system, whereby personal objectives and outcomes, or quality of life measures, are recorded and monitored over time. Perhaps you've elected to use an objective measure, such as return to work within a set time period following the completion of intervention. For information on suitable tools to use for outcome measurement, RCSLT have compiled details on a range of outcome measurement tools and systems that are in current use within the SLT profession (see Resources for web address). These outcomes can be systematically reported, either from previous client records (retrospective) or from discussions with future clients (prospective). Table 8.4 provides an example of a data record for adults with dysphonia, with return to work being the outcome measure used.

Table 8.4: Sample Data Collection Record for Q3 - How many adults with dysphonia return to work?

	Same employment	Different employment	Total
Return to full time work	20	5	25
Return to part time work	10	15	25
Unable to return to work	5	Not applicable	5
Total	35	20	55

Data analysis

Much of the analysis required for the type of data collected in relation to the question, 'how many clients do I have that ...' is quantitative analysis, dealing with numbers. The initial analysis will be in the form of percentages. For example, for Table 8.2, where the data shows the nature of presentation and its severity, each 'box' can be reported as a simple figure, as the percentage of the presentation or the severity, and as an overall percentage of the total sample, as shown in Table 8.5.

Table 8.5: Presentation and severity percentages.

	Receptive Expressive (RE)	Expressive only (E)	Total
Mild	N=100 %RE=100/500=20% %Mild=100/150=67% %Total=100/700=14%	N=50 %E=50/200=25% %Mild=50/150=33% %Total=50/700=7%	N=150 %Total=150/700=21%
Moderate	N=250 %RE=250/500=50% %Mod=250/325=77% %Total=250/700=36%	N=75 %E=75/200=38% %Mod=75/325=23% %Total=75/700=11%	N=325 %Total=325/700=46%
Severe	N=150 %RE=150/500=30% %Severe=150/225=67% %Total=150/700=21%	N=75 %E=75/200=38% %Severe=75/225=33% %Total=75/700=11%	N=225 %Total225/700=32%
Total	N=500 %Total=500/700=71%	N=200 %Total=200/700=29%	N=700 100%

If you have identified the number of referrals, divided into specific categories, for example months, you will have a series of 12 data sets. From this, you could identify the average, or mean, number of referrals each month. This involves dividing the total figure by the number of categories to find the average. For the example above, of 700 referrals, the mean would be 700/12, that is, 58 per month. You can then report the fluctuation across the year, not only numerically, but also as being above or below the mean and by how much.

Calculation of the mean does not consider any exceptional findings, for example a month with unusually high or low referrals. A better measure could be the median, or middle of your range. For this, place all your values in ascending value, and identify the middle value; where you have an even number, take an average of the middle two values in the line. More information and practice at calculating the mean, median and mode is available in Hinton (2004).

There are many other statistical calculations that can be carried out on your final data set. Rather than replicate all here, the reader is advised to refer to one of the many reference books available; see Further Reading for suggestions.

An alternative would be to meet with a local statistician, who is available in many of the support networks discussed earlier in this chapter.

Potential reporting framework

Whilst every report produced will have a different slant, depending on its nature and its intended audience, there are a few standard elements which are good practice to include. Examples of sections relating to the three questions posed above are provided within the sample framework below.

Context

It is essential that the scene is set, outlining the nature of the service and the locality in which it is provided, together with a summary of the local population data, available from census data from the Office of National Statistics (see Resources at the end of the chapter). It may also be helpful to provide a brief narrative about the service or section to which the report relates, summarizing the history (for example, this service has been established for n years).

Defining the question

It is important that a summary of the purpose of the report is provided, including the key question or questions that are being addressed.

Background/Introduction/Relevant literature

This is where you set out the key literature relating to your question. Be as precise and specific as you can, but ensure that your literature summary explains any technical jargon that you use, whether in your text or in any quotations that you use. It is often worth asking someone from outside of the profession to read this section, to ensure that you have explained all necessary terms.

For example, as well as the obvious technical terms such as 'aphasia' or 'SLI', we often use terms such as 'review' or 'intensive' which seem obvious to us but the reader might not understand.

If your professional body has produced evidence-based documents relating to your field or question, consider including relevant quotes, as this gives your reader the context of minimum standards of service delivery and so on, and provides a benchmark with which you can make comparisons from your findings.

It is helpful to add in references to key literature that support your report and its findings. These could be about the general population and incidence or prevalence estimates or comments about the socio-economic distribution and the implications for speech, language and communication needs or swallowing and feeding difficulties.

Be as selective as you can here; you are providing a brief context, not a thesis chapter, so aim to be as concise as you can, selecting only the most relevant references.

Data collection

Consider how you will specify and report your methods so that there is transparency. This may be as simple as saying something like, 'This data was collected from existing sources, relating to the last six months and the findings have been extrapolated from there. This provides a very good estimate of future needs, but minimal variation cannot be excluded as a possibility'.

Findings/results/main report

In planning this main section, consider the following:

- What are your key messages?

- Why are your results important?

- What action should be taken?

An example that summarizes the potential report content relating to the third of the three hypothetical questions used throughout this chapter is given below. Please note that the recommendations and conclusions are for example purposes only and do not necessarily reflect the current evidence base.

> *How successful is the service you offer?*
> (Example relating to the final hypothetical population, adults with dysphonia?)
>
> The ultimate objective of working with adults with dysphonia of such severity that it prevents them from attending work, is to remediate them sufficiently to return to the workplace, be this their original profession – the ideal – or an alternative job role – the compromise position.
>
> During the past x months, we have received 55 referrals of adults with dysphonia which have had such an impact. Of these, we have successfully returned 50 (91%) to employment of some sort.
>
> 27 (54%) returned to their prior post, 20 of which were full-time roles; a further 3 (6%) managed to return to their prior role with a reduction in their hours.
>
> A further 20 (40%) returned to employment in a different role, and 8 (16%) also reduced their hours.
>
> All but 3 of those who returned to some form of employment reported that they were pleased with that as an outcome of their intervention.

Implications and conclusions

These should be to the point but, dependent on your audience, can be quite far reaching as long as you are true to the evidence base, whether published or your own practice-based evidence. Ensure that your concluding statement is clear and concise, and fits the brief for your main audience. You could consider providing conclusions with different slants if you plan to send your report to a variety of readers, so that it is targeted to each of their interests and purposes.

An example conclusion for the sample report given above could be as follows:

> The approach we use for clients with voice difficulties has
> been proven effective, based on client satisfaction and the
> outcome of return to employment. The small proportion

who were unable to return to work had complex issues which will take more time to resolve. We therefore intend to continue this service delivery model.

Summary

You hold the key to a vast amount of clinical information, in paper and electronic form, and with a little organization and some time, you can collate this information to answer a range of questions and provide an array of reports. Evaluating information that you already possess does not require ethical approval, but it is worth liaising with your organization's Research and Development (R&D) department lead to obtain agreement for a retrospective service evaluation.

It is equally possible to undertake prospective service evaluation, provided you are specific about both the question or questions you want to ask and the information you require. Again, your R&D lead can offer support here. Whichever you choose to do, or if you choose a combination of the two approaches, set up a simple database or spreadsheet on which to record your findings as you go, since this will ease your statistical analysis later.

Remember that your clients and their families are a rich source of information, and should be consulted on the success of your service and on its future reorganization. It is important to target your questions so that you ask about those issues of direct relevance to them; that way, you receive informed comments and suggestions, as well as having the opportunity to obtain information about how satisfied they are with the service they have received to date. There is a range of means of collecting their wishes, levels of satisfaction, expectations and aspirations, and you will reap the benefits from their involvement. Finally, enjoy! This is your service, your team, your responsibility and your vision for the future. Undertaking service evaluation, whether retrospective or prospective or a combination, helps everyone to clearly see where the service currently sits and how it can develop in the future, securing funding, contracts, clientele, staff. It ensures that you provide a model of service delivery that is fit for purpose, fits with the evidence base and meets the wishes of the funding bodies and the population at large.

References

Enderby, P., John, A., & Petheram, B. (2006) *Therapy Outcome Measures for Rehabilitation Professionals: Speech and Language Therapy, Physiotherapy, Occupational Therapy* (2nd edition). Chichester: John Wiley & Sons.

Hinton, P. (2004) *Statistics Explained*. Hove: Routledge.

McLeod, S.M. & Threats, T. (2008) The ICF-CY and children with communication disabilities. *International Journal of Speech-Language Pathology* **10:1–2**, 92–109.

Threats, T. (2006) Towards an international framework for communication disorders: Use of the ICF. *Journal of Communication Disorders* **39:4**, 251–265.

Further reading

Hickson, M. (2008) *Research Handbook for Health Care Professionals*. Chichester: John Wiley & Sons.

Lowe, D. (1993) *Planning for Medical Research: A Practical Guide to Research Methods*. Congleton: Astraglobe Ltd.

Pring, T. (2005) *Research Methods in Communication Disorders*. London: Whurr.

Resources

American Speech and Hearing Association for best evidence summaries. http://www.asha.org

Office of National Statistics website for information on the local population: http://www.ons.org

RCSLT (2009). Resource Manual for Commissioning and Planning Services. Available at www.rcslt.org/speech_and_language_therapy/commissioning/resource_manual_for_commissioning_and_planning_services

RCSLT (2010) The Matrix Report. Available at www.rcslt.org/matrix_report

RCSLT (2011) Speech and Language Therapy Clinical Outcome Measurement Tools or Systems. Available at www.rcslt.org/members/outcome_measurement_tools

SpeechBITE for best evidence summaries: http://www.speechbite.com

Part III Next steps

9 Sharing your findings

Rosemarie Hayhow

Learning outcomes

By the end of this chapter, you will:

- Understand the importance of disseminating research findings
- Be able to write a dissemination plan
- Know how to proceed with a range of dissemination mediums and audiences
- Be able to identify specific additional support or guidance required to facilitate appropriate dissemination

---

Introduction

In this chapter, we consider the different ways in which the results from your study can be shared. Ideally, you will have developed a dissemination plan when you were writing your protocol. With more formal research studies this is an essential part of planning and contributes to the justifications for funding, time off work, research degree, etc. With a smaller piece of work, we may be less confident of obtaining useful results and so can find it difficult to work out a detailed dissemination plan prior to starting the study. The importance of a well-constructed dissemination plan is often not given sufficient weight and yet, without appropriate sharing of findings, the potential value of the study is not fulfilled. In addition, inadequate dissemination can lead to the needless replication of studies and so fail to satisfy one of the basic criteria of good, ethical research: that it contributes in some way to our collective understanding or knowledge and so influences our practice.

One of the common reasons for insufficient dissemination is lack of time and it is essential that practitioner-researchers make full use of all resources available to them to facilitate the process. This chapter aims to elaborate the steps in the process of dissemination and to indicate some of the available resources, bearing in mind that new and better resources could become available at any time. Completion of this stage can make a difference to practice, can motivate further professional development and inspire others to take up the challenge of contributing to the evidence base. Conversely, as Silcock warns (2009) in his presentation,

> "No matter how successful the research, improvements in care will only follow if the findings are communicated to the relevant people" (slide 5).

There are different ways of thinking about the dissemination process, but all involve an exploration of options and perusal of the materials associated with the particular newsletter, journal, magazine, website, meetings, etc., that you might target. This helps you identify the audience and medium or publication most likely to be interested in your work and their specific contributor requirements.

In the first section of this chapter the stages in the development of a dissemination plan are discussed (see Figure 9.1) and possible actions identified. The following section discusses ways of disseminating your findings and also identifies some resources and guidance that can help with the practicalities of sharing your work.

The dissemination plan

The aim of this section is to clarify the steps that will help you decide how to disseminate your findings. These steps, summarized in Figure 9.1, can also be considered when planning a project, so that you can include a dissemination plan in your proposal and identify any additional training or support that you require.

What have you found out?

Purpose: The purpose of this stage in the dissemination plan is to describe what you have found out in as succinct a manner as possible. This involves stripping away the trends, the implications and other thoughts you might have had during your analysis and interpretation of your data and focusing on the nub of what you have learned and the evidence you have for it.

Actions: Write down your primary finding or, in a qualitative study, write down your major themes and any subsidiary themes.

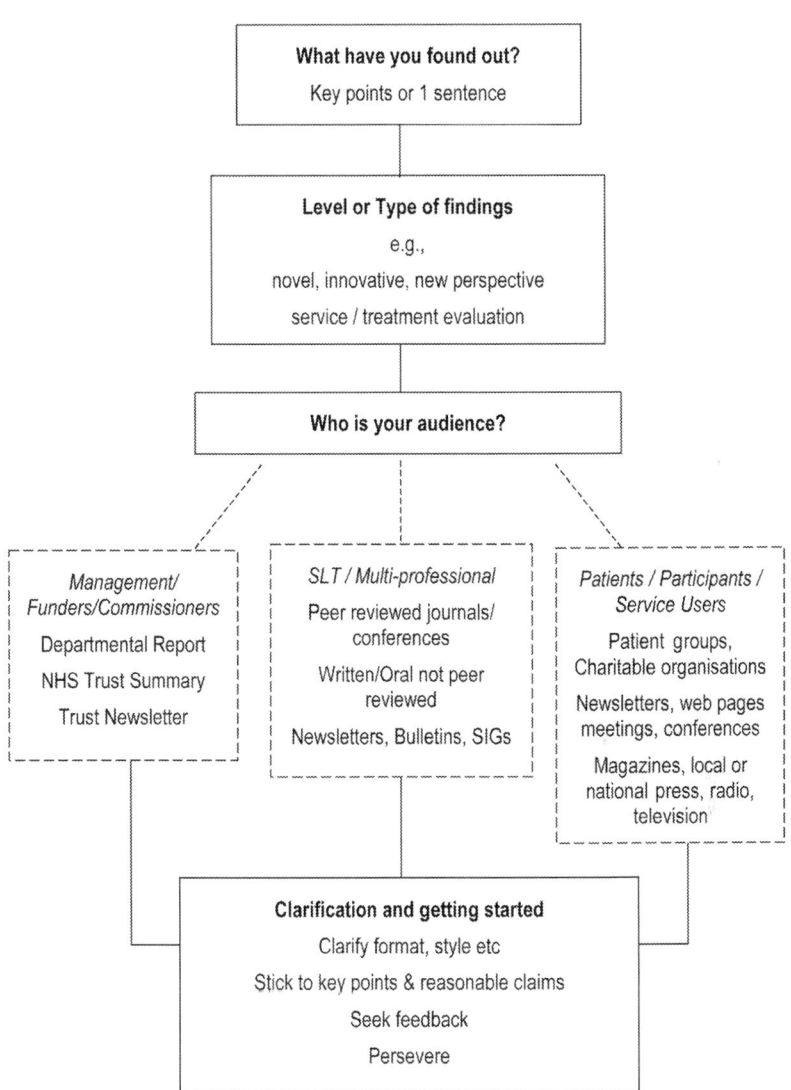

Figure 9.1 Summary of steps in dissemination plan.

Now we will consider the steps identified in Figure 9.1

Write a sentence that includes your main finding and that would get somebody interested in your study. If they respond well to this, what would you say next to keep their interest? This task was posed by one of my PhD supervisors. After the initial shock of being asked to reduce all my hours of work into one sentence, I could see that the task was sharpening my focus on what I had found out and making me think in lay terms about my findings; no waffle or hiding behind jargon. This exercise also helps you to steer away from false or over-optimistic claims.

Level or type of findings

Purpose: Knowing what level or type of findings your research has generated will guide you in your choices of where and what to disseminate. In your initial study design, you gave careful thought to your research question and the sort of data or information that were needed to answer it. Your review of previous work will have helped you identify whether your study is innovative and expanding the knowledge base, or whether it is more focused on your particular service and the ways in which the existing materials, knowledge and resources are used. Work that expands the knowledge base could be suitable for conferences and peer review journals, as well as for more local dissemination. Even modest findings can be worth sharing, as they could stimulate further research or, when combined with published research, add to an emerging picture. In the research and academic worlds, dissemination is primarily targeted at high impact peer review journals and funders require dissemination at this level as endorsement of the study. Smaller studies could be appropriate for clinically focused journals, newsletters or bulletins (professional and user groups), local radio or websites.

A focus on local service delivery issues does not necessarily preclude wider dissemination. For example, if the findings were unexpected and led you to reconsider some of the assumptions held about a client group or an intervention, then what started as a service evaluation takes on a broader significance. Decisions concerning the level or type of study and findings need not be taken alone. Someone looking at your study from the outside could appreciate its significance in a way that is lost to you, as familiarity can lead to an underestimation of the value of your work. It can happen the other way round, where the extent of your effort makes you feel your findings must be useful, but to an experienced, outside eye it looks like more of the same. It is important to get this worked out before you waste time on pursuing dissemination in a context where it will be refused. However, remember that even experienced researchers have articles refused and that the ratio between accepted and rejected articles varies between journals.

When a study is small, or where results are inconclusive, it does not mean there is nothing to share. It may be appropriate to share your experiences so that others can learn from it and so your work becomes a building block. In this instance, special interest groups (SIGs), Royal College of Speech and Language Therapists (RCSLT) *Bulletin* and user group newsletters would all be appropriate targets. It might be more difficult to publish negative or inconclusive results because of dissemination and publication biases (Song, Parekh, Hooper, Loke, Ryder, Sutton, et al., 2010) and yet rigorous researchers and practitioners value these, as they could save further wasted effort into unproductive areas.

When considering the 'level' of a research study it is important not to equate sample size with the value of the study. Small studies can be an important first step in developing a programme of research. For example, Phase I studies (Pocock, 1996) investigate whether the treatment has a therapeutic effect on a small number of participants and can lead to Phase II. Phase II studies still involve small numbers of participants and could include, among other things, a refinement of the treatment protocol, a further investigation of the size and consistency of the treatment effects or unwanted or unexpected treatment effects. These Phases prepare the ground for Phase III, or randomized controlled trials (RCT). These research phases have been related to communication impairment by Robey and Schultz (1998). In a further discussion of the phases, Robey (2004) indicates how this framework can be used to assess the thoroughness of published research and so is helpful reading in the early stages of your study design.

Actions: Be clear about your findings and think about what they mean and how they fit into the existing knowledge base. Think also about the scientific rigour of your study; a small and well-constructed study will have an audience whereas a large but badly-designed one will not.

You are now in a position to think about who your audience might be and where they might access their information.

Who is your audience?

Purpose: This stage will help you identify your potential audience so that you clarify who might want to know about your research findings, who needs to know and who you would like to inform. Figure 9.1 identifies three categories of people who might have an interest in your work and each needs information tailored to their context and specific requirements. In many cases, you will need to communicate with each group, but the scale of the study, strength of your findings and where it sits in relation to previous or further studies will influence the length and comprehensiveness of your reports or other feedback.

You will be required to report back to anyone who has supported your study in any way and there could be others who might benefit from learning about your work. Your enthusiasm for sharing what you have learned will be tempered by the time and money available for dissemination. If you think your study could be accepted as a conference poster or paper you may need to approach managers and research support services for extra funding to cover some of the costs this would entail. Professional bodies sometimes have a conference budget for which any members can apply, and there might be other local or charitable sources of funding that your research support team can advise you about. Writing peer-reviewed journal articles can be time consuming but there is considerable variation from one journal to another with regard to the length of article they accept. Only you can judge what is feasible if you need to write in your own time or have limited support.

Actions: List everyone who has been involved in your study and beside their names write their role and the aspects of your study that they would find particularly interesting. Think about your findings and whether they will be of interest to a wider audience. Now put each of the people you have identified into one of the groups in Figure 9.1 (managers; professionals; patients and participants) so that you are ready to think more specifically about how you will communicate with them.

For convenience, we will think about the three groups of people listed in the subheading as distinct, but there is overlap and individual circumstances will vary. The aim of this section is to identify some of the possible audiences and the most usual mediums for communication and so provide a framework to guide the dissemination process. Any dissemination is likely to include four areas: why, how, what you found, and what it means. The level of detail, the selected medium, the language, writing style, etc. will vary according to your audience and to the conventions that apply to that particular type of dissemination.

Management, funding bodies and service level dissemination

Purpose: There are three things to consider that might be relevant to your study: accountability, reaching the decision-makers and kudos. Any time away from your usual work, or time spent in research that you do as part of your job and any financial support you receive need to be accounted for. You might have kept a log of your research activities and you will have research files containing all your study documentation and data. These are an important part of your research accountability. You will also need to write a report at the end of your study, or possibly complete a form, so that results and completion are systematically recorded for whoever provided financial or other support. You might not have completed everything at this stage, but would be expected to indicate any outstanding work you intend to do. The length and level of detail of such reports vary so you will need to follow specific guidelines. You will also be required to write a concluding report for the ethics committee that approved your study and for your Research and Development (or Innovation) department, using the templates that they provide.

Colleagues who work with the same patient or client group will have an interest in hearing about your study in a less formal way. This could be done through a regular newsletter as well as face-to-face in small groups. Employers benefit from research-active staff and usually want research findings communicated as widely as appropriate. If your findings have the potential to reduce costs without compromising levels of care, the publicity department may also be interested in wider publication. If your study suggests that an aspect of current practice within your department needs changing, then you will need to write a report for your manager that shows your evidence and the rationale for suggested changes to practice. Ideally, these adaptations should then be the focus of a further study to see if the changes are beneficial.

Action: Identify the type of feedback or report that is required by your management, discuss this with your line manager and also talk about how you should disseminate your research to colleagues. If you do not have forms to complete or guidelines for report writing, then look at some previously-written reports or templates from other funding bodies or management. If you have some structure for your report it will make writing much easier. Refer back to your list of involved and potentially interested people and separate out those with whom you have a work connection. Consider staff meetings, training events or newsletters as possible contexts for communication.

Speech and language therapy or multi-professional

Purpose: Often the primary purpose in communicating our research with colleagues beyond our immediate work circle is to improve practice in some way. Systematic hypothesis testing is one way of gradually improving practice, where each small-scale study adds to our understanding. Wider dissemination through Specific Interest Groups (SIGs), newsletters, etc. can encourage others to build on your study. This accumulation of knowledge can be part of an iterative approach which helps us unpick those aspects of a complex intervention that are active treatment components (Medical Research Council, 2008).

Action: Here we focus on dissemination with speech and language therapy (SLT) colleagues, but the process is much the same when your work is more appropriately shared with members of a multidisciplinary team. From your list of interested people, identify the professionals and peers. For example, if you decide that your primary audience is SLTs working with similar client groups, then consider whether your work is at a level likely to be acceptable to a peer review journal. The journal web pages will guide you and help you consider whether your potential paper fits best with a journal that accepts articles across a wide range of client groups or would suit an impairment specific journal. Find out the dates and themes of potential conferences. If you feel your work is of interest, but not at this level then SIG meetings, bulletins or newsletters could be the right context.

Patients, participants and service users.

Purpose: There are different reasons for disseminating research findings directly to the people who are on the receiving end of our services. We need to conduct research that users will find relevant and acceptable and we need participants for our studies. Relationships between professionals and patients/clients/users have become increasingly reciprocal with many people wanting to be better informed about research and new findings. Charitable organizations with a focus upon communication and communication impairment fund research and provide information for their members. In some cases, they have the capacity to reach a wider range of people than we can through their newsletters, web pages and blogs. They may also use social networking sites, or organize support and self-help groups and conferences where users and professionals come together. People we work with also read newspapers and magazines, listen to the radio and watch television. Our task is to find the appropriate mediums for our findings.

Action: Discuss with your service user contacts the best way forward and consider what and how you will share with your participants. Compared with dissemination to peers, you can make fewer assumptions about educational level, preferred mediums for seeking information and understanding of vocabulary and concepts. Refer back to your list of people who might be interested and you should now just be left with those who fall into this group. A mind map (Buzan, 2002) is one way to think about this possibly diverse group and their preferred ways of accessing information. Consider age, education, level of understanding about the specific treatment or communication problem and other factors that could influence what they might want to know and how best to share this.

Clarification and getting started

Purpose: You have summarized the why, how and what of your study, your key message(s), and identified your target audience(s): now you must do the necessary research to ensure that what you write or prepare will be acceptable to that audience.

Actions: What follows is indicative rather than exhaustive:

- **Written dissemination**: Look at author guidelines for your target publication; these can be viewed on the publication website. If you are aiming for a less formal publication look at back copies of the target and identify the style, voice, vocabulary and length, etc. of the articles. If you need to write a report, look at some current reports for this audience and use these as a template for yours.

- **Verbal dissemination**: Think about the people, the contexts or environment where it will take place, the time frame and the best ways of supporting your verbal content. Think also about how you will modify your message and delivery for different audiences, for example, SIG group versus user feedback.

Whatever your chosen audience and medium, reflect upon your experiences of being on the receiving end of others' dissemination. Make a list of the pitfalls you want to avoid and how you will circumvent them. Use the internet, your NHS library, colleagues and any other resources you can think of that will help you clarify how you will proceed. Although you should expect to edit whatever you write or prepare, you will save yourself time by good planning in the early stages.

We now move away from Figure 9.1 and think further about the process of dissemination and where support can be obtained. Our main focus is upon dissemination to other professionals as this is arguably the most demanding option and the process and skills required are relevant to other audiences.

Types of dissemination

This section starts with a discussion of conference presentations, then writing an abstract, poster preparation, oral presentation and, finally, general and scientific writing tips. Much of the process is the same for less formal presentations and writing, so even if you do not intend to disseminate at conferences or write a journal article, selective reading of this section should still be helpful.

Conference presentations

The first steps with conference presentations are the same as for any form of dissemination. You must consider the question: what have I got to say and who will be interested in hearing it? Once you have identified your target conference you will need to look carefully at the presentation options and the guidelines for each of these. The sort of material that is suited to short presentations is different to a workshop. The former is often a research report while the latter is more directly relevant to clinical work and may involve: teaching new skills; using existing skills within a new framework; or demonstrating therapy procedures that are not usually used with the specific client group. Generally, workshops encourage interaction, whereas presentations are didactic with allocated questions and answer time at the end.

Occasionally, conferences have only poster presentations but more often there are designated time slots for posters. It is useful to find out how important poster sessions are in a particular conference before opting for this format. When posters are valued they are given plenty of time and are located within large areas where people will be able to browse and talk with the authors.

When poster sessions are tagged on at the end of a morning or afternoon and are located within the circulation space they can be dissatisfying for all. Properly organized poster sessions can be stimulating and facilitate more useful discussion than occurs within the time constraints of a 20-minute presentation. Conference presenters and participants who are less confident could find posters a good introduction to conferences.

Whether you opt for a poster, a paper, or a workshop you will have to write an abstract that will be reviewed by the conference scientific committee or review panel. They will accept, maybe conditionally, or decline your abstract or, alternatively, they might suggest a different format to the one you have identified as being best suited to your material. The requirements for the abstract, poster or power point presentation are much the same, regardless of whether it is a professionals' conference or users' conference or some other sort of meeting. The content must be tailored to the audience. To capture and maintain the interest of our audiences, materials need to be well-structured and presented. In addition, they must be of interest to the audience and delivered in a manner that takes account of their particular perspective, age, circumstances strengths and difficulties.

The abstract

All conference submissions require an abstract and guidelines are given which must be adhered to. Failure to follow the guidelines could lead to rejection even if your content looks relevant. Relevance is an important issue when writing for any audience or context and it is your responsibility to indicate how your work is relevant. The abstract is the basis for the acceptance or rejection of presentations and also written for your potential audience. You want them to be sufficiently interested in your work to choose to listen to you rather than to someone else. However, accuracy is also important, as you do not want people to leave your presentation halfway through when they realize it is not what they expected. When you write an abstract for a journal article you will probably complete this once you have written the article but with conferences the abstract could be written first. Usually abstracts are required several months before the conference and if the relevant conference happens only every two to three years, you may need to write your abstract while you are still analyzing your data in preference to waiting for the next opportunity.

The primary audiences for your abstract are the review panel, conference delegates or potential readers; however it is useful to think of others who might also read it. Albarran (2007) suggests a third audience comprizing the media, journal editors and user or patient groups who will approach your abstract with a different knowledge base. As with any writing, remember your target audience and try to put yourself in their shoes as you read the drafts of your abstract. The shorter the required summary of your work, the more carefully you have to choose your words and Lindquist (1993 cited in Albarran, 2007) recommends the three 'Rs' to keep the writer focused, namely *reducing, refining* and *reviewing* (p. 572).

The structure of your abstract mirrors the structure of your presentation or article and usually includes the following:

- A short title that clearly indicates your topic

- An introduction or background that identifies the problem and leads to the aims of your investigation

- An outline of the methods and procedures that you used, followed by a summary of your results or the trends in your initial analysis, if analysis is not yet complete

- The limitations of your study followed by conclusions and then the implications for practice

- Finally, any study you do, no matter how small, should be conducted in an ethical manner and in some contexts it is required that you make explicit the procedures you followed to safeguard your participants.

It is also worth remembering that conducting a study is a process and that by the time we get to writing-up, even a small piece of work, we have probably forgotten what we didn't know at the outset and this can lead us to make assumptions about the level of knowledge of our potential readers. This is when a colleague who is less familiar with your work can be a helpful reviewer.

The acceptance of your abstract gives the go ahead for the next stage which will be writing or developing a poster, a presentation or a workshop.

Posters

Much of what applies to an abstract also applies to a poster. Although you can give more information than in an abstract, you will still need to attend to the three 'Rs' (*reducing, refining* and *reviewing*). A good first step is to clarify why you are presenting a poster and what you want your take-home message to be.

You can then think about the best ways to convey this. In addition to text, will you use pictures, graphs, quotations from participants or cartoon type drawings? How these relate to your text and fit in with the overall design of your poster also needs consideration. There will be criteria set by the conference and these must be adhered to but you could also have considerable freedom. Effective posters have a balance between text and graphics and avoid unnecessary visual distractions. If you design your poster to stimulate your reader you are more likely to have interesting questions to discuss during your poster session.

Where you have your poster printed will influence design and cost, which in turn could influence the number of colours you can use. The amount of design help that is part of the printing service will vary, as will their experience with different sorts of studies and audiences. Most NHS hospital trusts have a medical illustration department with experience in designing and printing posters for health-related conferences. Discussion with colleagues should help identify the pros and cons of using the support services available to you and suggest how these compare with your local printers.

Pontin and Albarran (2008) give practical guidance on preparing conference posters, including layout, design and content and they suggest a poster needs to be read in less than ten minutes. It can be helpful to have an A4 handout version to give to interested delegates. If you choose to do this, then you need to design a poster that is still readable and pleasing to look at when reduced to one or two sides of A4.

Oral presentations

Your presentation slides should support your verbal content by orientating your audience to the key points and helping them engage with your topic. When slides are well planned and visually attractive, they take some of the pressure off the speaker by dividing the visual attention, emphasizing key points and keeping the speaker on track.

There are tutorials and guidelines on slide design. A good example is available from the website of the International Association of Science and Technology for Development (see Resources). Their tips are presented on *Power point* slides so you see what a good colour scheme, font size, organization, etc., look like in contrast to the slides where these things are less reader-friendly. Bear in mind, your employer may have a slide template that you need to use and don't forget to include acknowledgements and contact details on your last slide.

Once you are happy with your slides you then need to work on the spoken component. Sometimes people read their presentation and, when time is short, this is a good way to avoid over-running or getting side-tracked. However, it is hard to engage with your audience if you are reading from your presenter notes or from a script. The ideal is to be so familiar with your material that you can speak from memory with your slides working as triggers. This requires confidence and a strict adherence to the timeframe you have worked out for your slides. Some versions of *PowerPoint* (Microsoft) or *Keynote* (Mac) have presenters' tools that help with timing and notes. It is worth rehearsing your presentation several times so that you know which slide you should be talking about at any particular time-point in your presentation. If you are including sound or video samples, or importing any other additional data, you must make sure this will work seamlessly. It is better to rely on description than incorporate videos where the sound won't play or add-ins that don't automatically fire up when you move to the relevant slide.

The ideal rehearsal is with supportive colleagues who will give you honest and helpful feedback. They can also ask questions so that you have some experience of thinking on your feet and giving appropriate answers. Presentations often last for around 15 minutes with five minutes for questions. You need not fear questions you cannot answer since you can compliment the questioner on their thought-provoking input. This might give you the time you need to formulate a response or, if it is outside your current area of competence, suggest you meet later to discuss the issue. Sometimes questioners try to take the floor and the presenter needs to regain control; when this is proving difficult, the chair of the session should come to your rescue. If they don't, you may need to be firm and politely move on to another question. The audience will usually be pleased that you have taken control in this way.

Workshops

Workshops are another format for sharing developments in clinical practice and could be an option at conferences or be the best format in other contexts where audience participation is desirable.

There is a range of potential workshops that could develop from a study, and your audience, their particular requirements and the information that will be relevant to them will again primarily influence the content and format. Workshops need a carefully crafted balance between the didactic and experiential components and small group discussions and feedback sessions need strict monitoring. A conference workshop will require an abstract that should give a clear indication of the content and what your workshop will entail, so that people get what they expect and are neither overwhelmed nor bored. If you are not familiar with your potential workshop participants, then you will need guidance from those with relevant experience.

If you are attempting an activity, demonstration or other novel procedure then you must rehearse this, maybe with colleagues, so that you can see if it works as you anticipated and if people learn from it as you expected. Workshops are longer than presentations and require meticulous planning if you are not an experienced educator. A well run workshop can be stimulating for participants and presenters and is an ideal context for sharing what you have learnt in your study and moving on to more practical issues.

What sort of study or findings could lend themselves to a workshop format? A general example might help answer this question. Suppose you conducted an interview study with a small number of relatives or carers of a particular client group and found recurring themes around feelings of *isolation from others in the same position, confusion about the aims of therapy sessions* and *frustration at not knowing how to help their relative in everyday communication*. These preliminary findings are worth sharing, even if they confirm what people might already suspect, as your research has moved them beyond anecdote and initiated the process of providing better care. Workshops could be the ideal context for sharing and further development. You might set up some relative/ carer workshops with the aim of finding out if these themes resonate with a larger audience. It is likely that they will, as you will have thought carefully about the sampling procedures for your study and probably invited a range of participants. The next aim of your workshop might be to develop some ideas about how these problems could be tackled. You might have some specific questions to explore, for example, what would make the therapy experience more relevant? How could feelings of isolation be reduced? What are the daily communication problems that leave relatives feeling inadequate? A workshop that combines sharing findings and developing better practice requires careful planning, not just to achieve the aims, but also to record the new information. You might like to enlist the help of a colleague to share the load.

A similar workshop could be set up for colleagues where you share your findings and then work together on ways of addressing the issues raised by your study. Colleagues may also be interested in the details of your methods or what you learned about conducting small-scale research in a clinical setting.

This could lead to discussion of further research within the department, covering research questions, methodology, the nuts and bolts of running a study and the development of outline protocols. The time you would need or the number of workshops required for such ambitious aims would depend upon staff experience and knowledge, which brings us back to the importance of knowing your audience and keeping them in mind during your workshop planning.

You will need to work out clear aims for each part of your workshop and develop resources such as summary sheets, questions for small group discussion, a written structure for feedback or whatever else will help you and your participants get the maximum benefit from the workshop. There is some freely available workshop guidance that you can download from the internet (for examples, see Resources/Further Reading at the end of the chapter) and although not relevant in their entirety, they contain many useful points that help in the planning process.

Developing your confidence

Finally, before we leave face-to-face presentations a few words about confidence. As experts in human communication we should be able to give good oral presentations. However, there is a lot at stake when we share our findings and even experienced presenters can feel nervous. Rehearsal presentations with peers provide opportunities for constructive feedback and a context to practise breathing and relaxation skills and to work on your verbal and non-verbal communication style. When I have felt particularly nervous, a common occurrence in my early working life with people who stammer, I have thought about what such a presentation would demand of someone who stammers. This has always shamed me into thinking along the lines that I have discussed with clients. For example, to think about the skills I have and to use them, to focus on breathing to steady myself, to ensure I have a good grounded stance and open posture and look upon the audience as colleagues, not enemies. If you have something interesting to say, are well prepared, use appropriate resources and communicate an interest in your findings, then the chances are your presentation will be well-received.

A possible side effect of conducting a study is that it makes you aware of how much more there is to learn about the topic or area of investigation. However, you know your work better than anyone else and this is what you are sharing. It is usual for presenters and writers to briefly overview the limitations of their study and, when possible, indicate how their findings can inform further work. This allows you to place your study within the context of other work and to show both its weaknesses and strengths. If a question or comment takes you outside your area of competence, you can acknowledge what you don't know. You are more likely to be criticized for a poor response than for an honest acknowledgement of your limitations. Finally, it is worth remembering that, however well you perform, you will probably feel you could have done better so it can be helpful to, silently, acknowledge this. We need people to share their work if knowledge and understanding are to grow and we need informed and critical discussions to identify potential next steps in this learning process.

Writing up a study

Organizing your study information

Over the last 15 years there has been a quiet revolution in how we obtain, store and access information. Paper and ink have given way to digital storage and instead of index cards we use electronic systems to keep track of what we have read and where it is stored. Note-taking no longer needs to involve writing out what we are reading, we can now copy and paste and then organize in different ways. Bibliographies can also be stored with reference management software and produced in whatever style is required by your target publication (see Chapter 3). Moreover, specific software has been developed to help with thought organization and planning for writing-up. A web search of 'mind maps' will reveal a variety of free and for-sale packages. You may, justifiably, argue that one small study does not warrant the time and effort required to learn to use such software. However, this might be just the context where time invested will have a good return. The discipline of organizing your literature for your current study could pay dividends when you come to write it up as well as providing the basis of a larger digital library for future use. NHS Trust librarians are able to help with the use of search engines and reference storage and might also be familiar with other web-based resources that can help with the practicalities of writing.

Writing: General considerations

The process of writing can sometimes show up weaknesses in one's use of punctuation or other aspects of grammar. Fortunately, there are web-based learning tools to help improve these writing skills. I have used The University of Bristol, Faculty of Arts, 'Improve your writing' resource (see Resources at the end of the chapter). It has explanations of the grammatical rules and exercises with feedback so you can test your ability to apply these rules. Although this resource has been prepared for arts students, much of it is relevant to good writing generally and so is helpful for informal reports, user group newsletters, etc., as well as for scientific writing.

Discussion with colleagues can be helpful for clarifying your thinking and for obtaining useful feedback. If you are aiming to inform fellow practitioners, then asking a few colleagues to read your work will give you their perspective. It is also helpful to get feedback from someone who has experience of writing and reviewing for peer-reviewed journals and who can critically evaluate the scientific merit of your paper as well as its accessibility and suitability for your target audience. Albarran and Pontin (2008) advise giving your critical reader a clear idea of what you are asking of them and that you also attach the author guidelines for the target journal. You will need to decide how much feedback is helpful; too much conflicting feedback can sap confidence and make the task seem unachievable. However, if you do not seek some objective views you could unwittingly submit an inadequately prepared piece of work that will be rejected.

I was once advised that my writing style made my reader work too hard and so risked losing their attention and interest. It was a salutary warning. We can make things easier for our readers by indicating what we plan to cover in a section, so that they can orientate themselves. Linking the main ideas with short bridging text makes the logic of the structure more transparent. This saves the reader the distraction of trying to hold several ideas in mind while working out where the author is taking them. It is useful to remember that well- structured writing doesn't hold surprises; you don't get a 'where did that come from?' experience when reading a well-constructed text.

Learn from your mistakes and try not to get disheartened. This can be hard when you are asked to edit a piece of writing that you have already worked on. However, it is better to have work to edit than to put off getting started as the process of writing can help clarify your thinking and so reduce the feelings of uncertainty. Whenever I have been advised to go over some work and, for example, reduce unnecessary words, shorten the sentences, only include what I have evidence for, clarify my terms, think of a structure or style that will be easier for a wider audience or justify a claim, then the resulting piece of work has been better and the extra work eventually worthwhile.

There are other tips for writing that occur over and over in guidelines for all types of audience:

- Time is well spent clarifying your content and the sequence in which you plan to write it. Once this is established your writing will flow more easily.

- Give yourself reasonable chunks of time for writing; don't expect to be able to pick up writing for a few minutes here and there.

- When you need to finish for the day stop at the end of a section **and then** write some quick notes about what you will do next. These notes will help you when you come back to the work as it will be easier for you to pick up where you left off.

- When returning to writing, avoid re-reading what you last wrote. Work on the next part and then review a larger chunk when you reach a logical endpoint.

- Find the best environment for you, somewhere you can concentrate and, as far as possible, be free from distractions.

- Avoid using jargon unless it is appropriate to your audience and clarifies your message.

- Always keep your target audience in mind when you write.

There is often a frustrating incubation period when you feel stuck and despair of ever getting the writing done. I have not found a way around this and now accept that I have to ruminate before I write. There is an advantage, some menial jobs get done while I ruminate and there is a huge sense of relief when at last my writing flows.

Some are more fluent with talking than writing and recording a discussion with a colleague about the work, why you did it, the primary findings and what these findings might mean can help generate that essential structure and key points. You can then work from the audio recording. Alternatively, you might consider using speech recognition software and talk rather than write the first draft of your paper. This software has improved enormously in the last few years. It is now cheaper, requires less training to consistently recognize individual speaking patterns and, provided you continue to train the software as you write, becomes increasingly accurate. It is also invaluable to anyone who is slow at typing, or has repetitive strain injury or other problems exacerbated by long spells at the computer keyboard.

Scientific writing style

Those more recently qualified will probably still be familiar with the requirements of scientific writing but if you have not written an essay or extended report for a while, a refresher might be useful. There are many on-line resources available with varying levels of detail. An excellent chapter on writing a scientific paper can be found on the USA Oxford University Press (OUP) website (see Resources at the end of the chapter). This chapter gives sound practical advice, for example: short declarative sentences are the easiest to write and the easiest to read, and they are usually clear. However, too many short sentences in a row can sound abrupt or monotonous. To add sentence variety, it is better to start with simple declarative sentences, some of which you can combine, than to start with long rambling sentences which you try to shorten.

Some other recommendations from this chapter are paraphrased below:

- Tense: simple past tense for statements of what you did or others have done; present tense for statements of fact; simple past and present can both be used for results, discussion and conclusion.

- Use the active voice, as it is shorter and more direct than the passive. 'I wrote the report' is active, whereas, 'the report was written by me' is in the less punchy passive voice.

- Use one word in preference to a phrase, for example, a *few* is better than a *small number*.

- Use gender-neutral language so that 'man' becomes 'people', unless all participants were male or female when gender specificity would be appropriate. Avoid 'him' or 'her' by using the plural 'them', although a few instances of 'his or her' are acceptable.

The above gives an indication of what is available in the OUP chapter and this or something similar is good reading for anyone who needs a refresher on writing skills. Another useful resource is provided by Albarran and Scholes (2005) who warn against the following errors:

> Four of the most common mistakes made include papers
> that are submitted without a clear and logical structure,
> failure to state the aims/purpose of the article, lack of
> in-depth review of the literature or conclusions that are
> disproportionate to the results from data analysis. Other
> reasons for papers not meeting the required standards are
> to do with literary style, which can be obscure, convoluted,
> clumsy and inaccessible. (p. 75)

These authors list requirements for journal articles that are common to most, while stressing the importance of following the house rules that can be found in the guidance for authors on the journal publisher's website. They also discuss issues of authorship and acknowledgement, how to submit a paper and what to do when you receive the reviewers' and editors' responses. Even accepted papers nearly always have conditions attached and the reviewers' and editors' comments and requests must be worked through systematically so that you can show exactly how you have addressed their concerns.

Special audiences

Our knowledge of language development and impairment should put us in a strong position when we write for audiences with receptive language difficulties, or for others who come from a wide range of educational backgrounds. We are used to modifying our spoken language and many of us are experienced in giving verbal explanations or presentations to clients and carers. Moreover, there is a growing interest in the experiences of the people with whom we work and in sharing information with them. People with aphasia are one client group whose particular needs, with regard to written information, have been explored. Indeed, two recent studies (Rose, Worrall, Hickson, & Hoffmann, 2011, 2012) found that people who have aphasia agreed on factors that affected their ease of reading. Among the barriers to reading everyday documents were: too much information and text; small font size; and lack of headings. Some facilitators were: clear headings; well set out and concise use of language; and content divided into clearly defined sections. Graphics increased interest, facilitated understanding, made the items quicker to read and more memorable. The guidelines presented in these articles have relevance beyond aphasia and are a good reference when modifying written or *PowerPoint* work for people with educational disadvantage or language impairment.

We need to refer to existing and developing author or presenter guidelines when sharing our study with participants or users of our SLT services. As people become increasingly active in managing their health needs online, we anticipate that further guidelines will become available.

Summary

This chapter has highlighted the importance of dissemination in ensuring that research findings ultimately influence practice. The dissemination plan will help you to clarify your different audiences and their interests and provide a structure to help you complete this final stage. It is vital that the target audience is kept in mind when preparing materials for dissemination, and in particular, that you consider the dissemination medium that will be most appropriate for them. There are many resources available to help you, including written and on-line materials. And finally, don't forget that your colleagues and networks can be a huge support and assist you in the execution of your dissemination plan.

References

Albarran, J. W. (2007) Planning, developing and writing an effective conference abstract. *British Journal of Cardiac Nursing* **2**, 570–572.

Albarran, J. W. & Pontin, D. (2008) Getting published in a peer-reviewed journal. *British Journal of Cardiac Nursing* **3**, 38–41.

Albarran, J. W. & Scholes, J. (2005) How to get published: Seven easy steps. *British Association of Critical Care Nurses, Nursing in Critical Care* **10**, 72–77.

Buzan, T. (2002) *How to Mind Map*. London: Harper Collins.

Medical Research Council (2008) *Developing and Evaluating Complex Interventions: New Guidance*. http://www.mrc.ac.uk/complexinterventionsguidance (issued 29 September 2008, 1st accessed January 2009).

Pocock, S. J. (1996) *Clinical Trials – A Practical Approach*. Chichester: John Wiley & Sons.

Pontin, D. & Albarran, J. (2008) Preparing a conference poster. *British Journal of Cardiac Nursing* **3**, 117–120.

Robey, R. R. (2004) A five-phase model for clinical-outcome research. *Journal of Communication Disorders* **37**, 401–411.

Robey, R. R. & Schultz, M. (1998) A model for conducting clinical-outcome research: An adaptation of the standard protocol for use in aphasiology. *Aphasiology* **12**, 787–810.

Rose, T., Worrall, L., Hickson, L., & Hoffmann, T. (2011) Aphasia friendly written health information: Content and design characteristics. *International Journal of Speech-Language Pathology* **13**, 335–347.

Rose, T., Worrall, L., Hickson, L., & Hoffmann, T. (2012) Guiding principles for printed education materials: Design preferences of people with aphasia. *International Journal of Speech-Language Pathology* **14**, 11–23.

Silcock, J. (2009) *Disseminating Research: Choosing How & Where to Publish*. Retrieved 9 July 2011, from http://www.rdinfo.org.uk/flowchart/Presentation.ppt

Song, F., Parekh, S., Hooper, L., Loke, Y. K., Ryder, J., Sutton, A, J., Hing, C., Kwok, C. S., Pang, C., & Harvey, I. (2010) Definitions of dissemination, publication and related biases. *Health Technology Assessment* **14:8,** doi:10.3310/hta14080, © 2010 Queen's Printer and Controller of HMSO.

Resources

Strategies for a dissemination plan and sample posters, fliers, etc. to illustrate how to communicate your key findings:

Yale Center for Clinical Investigation, Community Alliance for Research and Engagement (CARE) *Beyond Scientific Publication: Strategies for Disseminating Research Findings*. Retrieved June 2011 from www.researchtoolkit.org/home/disseminating-and-closing-research/disseminating-and-measuring-impact.html

For information on preparing slides:

International Association of Science and Technology for Development

www.iasted.org/conferences/formatting/Presentations-Tips.ppt

For guidance on planning and preparing workshops:

Tiberius, R. & Silver, I. (2001) *Guidelines for Conducting Workshops and Seminars that Actively Engage Participants*. Retrieved 7 November 2011 from www.siumed.edu/resaffairs/documents/Conductingworkshops.doc

www.networklearning.org

For help with grammar and sentence structure:

Bristol University: http://www.bristol.ac.uk/arts/exercises/grammar/grammar_tutorial

For help writing scientific papers:

Oxford University Press: http://www.oup.com/us/samplechapters/0841234620/?view=usa#START

10 Moving on

Hazel Roddam

Learning outcomes

By the end of this chapter, you will know more about:

- The range of research degrees and how they differ
- What to expect as a postgraduate research student
- Sources of funding for your research ideas
- Getting support for research in the workplace
- Wider research networks
- How to network and make links with other research-active colleagues

---

Introduction

This chapter is written for therapists who have decided that they want to find a way to be research-active in the years ahead. Whatever the stage of your career, the aim is to help you to reflect on the previous chapters, and to build your own personal action plan for how you can start to achieve this ambition.

The chapter is laid out in three sections. The first section starts with a discussion of the relevant issues to consider before deciding whether you might want to enrol for a research degree, either at Masters or at Doctoral level. This includes reflecting on your personal circumstances, choosing the right degree and approaching potential supervisors. It then gives information about the range of academic routes and offers comments on the experience of undertaking a research degree. The second section covers a broad overview of funding options that you may be able to bid for: for paying enrolment fees and also for practice-based research project costs. The third section in this chapter gives advice on finding support for your research activities within your workplace and wider afield. Most importantly, this chapter aims to highlight the value of networking and making useful contacts for the future. You shouldn't plan to undertake research alone – and you don't need to.

Should I consider a research degree?

Many people make an assumption that before you can start to 'do research' you need to have a PhD. That is most certainly not the case. In fact, the aim of this book is encourage you to recognize that you already have a lot of relevant and transferrable skills to be a successful practitioner-researcher. However, you may feel that now is a good time to investigate the range of options for undertaking some formal training in research skills. These, for example, could be through attending Masters level modules, or through other professional development or research interest groups like the ones described later in this chapter. Training and support is also available through NHS Research and Development (R&D) departments, so it is valuable to find out what you can access there first.

However, for some people, the feeling that you have a personal goal to achieve a Masters or Doctoral degree just won't go away, so you may indeed decide to go ahead to enrol for a research degree. It is essential that you are certain that this is the right moment to embark on an academic course which will require a commitment of sustained effort over an extended period of time, and you need to feel confident that this is the right time in view of your work-life balance and other personal circumstances. This is the time to find out what support you would have to help you throughout your study, in your workplace and at home. Later in this chapter you will find some recommendations about accessing support from your manager and colleagues, as well as engaging in wider research networks.

This section of the chapter aims to explain the different academic routes and awards to help you decide whether any of these are right for you. National standards for registration of postgraduate research students are published in the Quality Assurance Agency (QAA) Code of Practice, to ensure that the highest possible academic standards are maintained, as well as promoting the most transparent assessment mechanisms (see Resources section at the end of the chapter for link). These standards include, for example, the minimum and maximum enrolment periods for full-time and part-time students and specifications for thesis lengths, to comply with the Higher Education Funding Council of England (HEFCE) regulations.

What type of degree should I choose?

Taught Masters courses

Across the UK there is a very large range of programmes at Masters level (MSc and MA), all of which will incorporate taught modules on research design, as well as a research-based dissertation or project. Some of these programmes are uni-professional routes which are specific to SLT. There are also a number of other programmes that have been explicitly developed to accommodate cross-discipline participation; one example of the latter would be a programme for practitioners from different backgrounds who work with children who have special educational needs. You may feel that the structure of a taught course would suit you well and help to focus your learning. Most of these Masters courses can be completed on either a full-time or part-time basis.

Alternatively, if you feel that you are ready to start thinking about practice-based research, then you might not want to invest the next two or three years as a part-time student to complete a full programme of module assignments, or to take a year out of employment to do the Masters on a full-time basis. Instead, you could consider simply enrolling for a single module, for example, an introduction to research design. If you have covered introductory-level research skills in your first degree, you might opt for a more advanced level module in a specific research approach that is particularly relevant to the methods for data collection or data analysis that you are planning to use. Modules are generally taught over one semester (approximately ten weeks). If you work in an NHS organization it is well worth checking whether there is a Service Level Agreement (SLA) in place with one of your local Higher Education Institutions (HEIs), which would cover the enrolment fee for the module. Some HEIs have also recently launched some distance-learning, e-learning and blended-learning options, which offer greater flexibility for many busy clinicians. If you work in the NHS it might be possible for you to undertake training sessions on these research skills within your own organization. The third section of this chapter includes further suggestions for optimising the support available from your local NHS R&D officers.

Research degrees

Undertaking a research degree is quite a different prospect from the classroom experience of a taught course, so it is particularly important to ensure that you have access to peer-group support as a postgraduate research student. Depending on where you enrol, there could be regular opportunities to meet other postgraduate research students. That gives the chance for mutual support and encouragement, so it's really important to enquire about this before you choose where to enrol. Hearing about other students' projects can also raise your awareness of alternative research designs and enhances your understanding of the research environment. Participation within an academic community helps you to keep up-to-date with research developments in broader areas than your own thesis topic and increases your confidence in academic debate (Lewis & Habershaw, 1997). For each of the research degree options below you would be assigned a supervisory team. The process of how research supervisors are allocated to students is discussed below to highlight a number of aspects that will be useful for you to consider.

Masters by Research (MRes)

A Masters by Research is a relatively small-scale piece of work that has the benefit of allowing first-time researchers to gain direct experience of the research process. As a full-time student you would expect to complete this in just over one year; as a part-time route it usually takes two years, although the national regulations allow for a maximum of three years. The dissertation is approximately 25,000 words. At the viva (oral examination), the candidate is expected to demonstrate a good understanding of relevant research approaches as well as to be able to present the findings of their study.

MPhil

The MPhil award has a slightly longer expected time-frame for completion than the MRes: up to three years full-time and up to five years part-time. The dissertation is also more substantial at 30,000–40,000 words. It is expected that the research design has a high level of academic rigour and that there will be in-depth analysis of the findings. If you register for the MPhil you need to be aware that it won't be possible to extend or transfer onto a PhD award at the end of your project, unless you have enrolled on the MPhil/PhD route described next.

MPhil/PhD

This award is increasingly being adopted by HEIs, rather than PhD Direct and there is some evidence that this process assists in increasing the rates of successful PhD completions. When you register your research proposal, the supervisory team will help you to define a transfer point which would be the equivalent of the MPhil level. The PhD component of the project might comprise additional data collection or, for example, be a proposal for a more in-depth analysis of the data, a synthesis with other theoretical frameworks, or the development of a conceptual model. At the transfer point you submit a report and might also have a viva. It may be that the university panel recommend an exit award at this point: they may do this if they have any concerns that either the candidate or the project do not have the potential to successfully achieve doctoral level. Hopefully, you will transfer smoothly and be ready to embark on the final phase of your project. With the agreement of your supervisory team you could request to submit a dissertation for an MPhil as an exit award at this point. You might want to do this for a wide range of personal reasons or changing circumstances, so the benefit to you as a student of enrolling on this route is evident.

PhD Direct

Many HEIs now only permit students to register on this route if they have recently completed a Masters by Research (MRes) and the proposal for their PhD project is a continuation of that work. In that case, the Masters-level research would serve as a feasibility or pilot study for the larger proposal. However in contrast with the MPhil/PhD route described above, the PhD Direct offers no alternative or early exit award, so you need to acknowledge that you could potentially end up with nothing to show for your work if you are not able to complete the PhD successfully for any reason. The guideline word limit for a PhD thesis is around 80,000 words. The regulatory timeframe for completion of a PhD is generally three to four years as a full-time student and six to seven years as a part-time student.

Professional Doctorate

There is an increasing number of Professional Doctorate programmes which are relevant for SLTs. The focus of a Professional Doctorate is explicitly on applied research in a workplace setting. It is expected that the research study will incorporate the implementation and evaluation of a practice-based change initiative within the student's own organization. The delivery of these programmes is generally on a part-time route, where the first two years comprise a number of taught modules. The modules are likely to include research design, management of organizational change and critical reasoning. At the end of the taught phase of the programme, each student is assigned a supervisory team and embarks on the research project element which will be approximately equivalent to the MPhil level described above. The Professional Doctorate could be of particular interest to SLTs who want to pursue a career route in management. If you think that you may potentially be interested in moving into an academic environment then it might be better to consider the traditional PhD route. If your primary aim is to continue in clinical practice in your specialist field, then either of these doctoral options could suit you, dependent on your own learning style and preferences for the way these programmes are structured.

What are the entry criteria for a research degree?

To register for a higher degree, most UK universities specify that you should have a good first degree, or 'equivalent experience'. You will be expected to assure your potential supervisors that you are seriously committed to pursuing this path, and are fully prepared to invest your own personal time throughout the period of the project, in addition to any time that your employer is prepared to allow you to use on your studies. They will also want to be convinced that you are not making this application on a whim; so any evidence you can provide to show that you have a sustained interest in research activities is important. And finally, do plan carefully about how you are going to present your outline ideas for your research question: you are not expected to have already prepared a detailed research design, but your prospective supervisors will look for indicators that you have a systematic problem-solving approach.

Once you have started as a postgraduate research student, you will undertake a programme of training in research skills in line with the UK Research Councils' best practice standards, as published on their website (see Resources at the end of the chapter). This statement specifies a requirement for students to have an awareness of the context of research as well as of research governance within their own discipline. These skills may be covered in a range of ways, including taught sessions, workshops, self-directed learning and supervisor support or mentoring. If it's been a while since you last undertook any academic study then it's highly likely that you'll need some additional support and skills development (Lewis & Habershaw, 1997). You may be unfamiliar and under-confident with current academic standards and conventions, so you'll need to discuss with your supervisors how you can most effectively update your knowledge and skills. This might incorporate basic study skills such as searching electronic databases and the management of electronic resources, critical appraisal of research designs, plus academic writing style, including referencing and awareness of plagiarism. In addition to research skills and techniques, you will also need to have skills in personal time management and effectiveness, project management, research management, personal effectiveness, communication skills, networking and team-working.

How does research supervision work?

Who will be part of the supervision team?

At most universities, you will have more than one academic supervisor: generally one subject specialist, plus another specialist in the relevant research methodology. The UK regulations require that at least one member of the team should have a minimum of two successfully completed supervisions, so that you can be assured that they are experienced in this role. All the team members should be research-active and have experience that is directly relevant to at least one aspect of the student's proposed work. There may be additional supervisors who have complementary expertise to offer. However, the nominated supervisory team will need to be confirmed by a university board, as a check that between them they are able to provide the range of support roles and discrete skills to match your project, and this should also have been discussed with you.

How do I choose the right supervisor?

From your perspective, your most important concerns are likely to be that your potential supervisors have the relevant experience and are also interested in your research project. You can expect to submit co-authored research papers with your supervisors and, after you've completed your degree, you may have the opportunity to continue working on research projects with them.

So when you start to consider where you might want to register it is worth spending time to look carefully at the research themes and publications of potential supervisors, to be as confident as possible that these resonate with your own perspectives about this aspect of your work. It is not essential that your supervisors are SLTs, provided that you think they have the most relevant experience for the project you will be working on. It is also likely that one or more of your supervisors may have limited direct experience of clinical practice contexts. However, whilst having clinical links might assist them to support you in recognizing how your clinical thinking skills relate to academic reasoning, you should not be disadvantaged provided that one of the team members has an awareness of clinical governance and professional issues within healthcare. Dependent upon your research field, there could also be external advisors who can be invited to contribute their input to the supervisory team, for example, clinical experts in the field.

Working with your supervisory team

Publications on theories of teaching and learning abound. To what extent these are directly relevant to the supervision of research students is moot, although there are doubtless many aspects of overlap and commonalities. The teaching of study skills and the facilitation of a student's critical thinking may be closest to the aims of supporting an individual to achieve academic independence at the appropriate level for a research degree award (Baxter Magolda, 1996). For you to be successful in gaining your target research award, you'll need to be able to demonstrate your progress in independent critical evaluation and academic thinking, both through your written thesis and your conduct in the viva examination. As a therapist, you already have strong skills in critical thinking and in problem-solving, and your supervisors will help you to progress in being able to successfully present your research arguments with appropriate academic rigour. You might find it useful to look at Bloom's model of critical thinking, which offers relevant constructs for identifying how an individual progresses towards higher level functioning (Bloom, 1956; Anderson & Krathwohl, 2001). Bloom's taxonomy identifies thinking skills of increasing cognitive complexity: encompassing knowledge, comprehension, application, analysis, synthesis and evaluation. As an experienced therapist, you will recognize direct parallels with recent conceptual modelling of the influences on therapists' clinical decision-making (Schon, 1983; van der Gaag & Anderson, 2005).

Roles and responsibilities of the supervisory team

The supervisory team will guide you to refine your research question and will ensure that you design a study that will be realistic and achievable, as well as academically robust. One of the principal functions of the supervisory team is to help you to develop increasing academic independence, towards the end point of submitting your thesis (Lewis & Habeshaw, 1997). Having a team of supervisors provides the opportunity for you to benefit from this range of expertise, but to function effectively as a team, it is important that all the members have explicitly agreed their respective roles within the group. You shouldn't expect that there will always be an exact consensus between the team; but this can give you realistic experience of academic debate. And it is your responsibility as the student for deciding how to act on the advice they give.

It is always recommended that you start out with an explicit agreement or contract regarding how the supervision arrangements are going to work. Throughout the period of your study it is your responsibility to prepare adequately for each supervision meeting. This includes attending the booked sessions, submitting drafts for your supervisors to read within the timescales agreed, and being prepared to respond to constructive criticism from the supervisory team. You have to take full responsibility for your own work and keep records of each meeting with your supervisors, so you will need to have good personal organizational skills. For their part, the supervisors' responsibilities include a commitment to giving their students uninterrupted time, giving constructive and detailed feedback on work submitted, and offering supportive advice to help the students to maintain their progress throughout their studies. The supervisors also keep a record of the meetings, plus other correspondence relating to specific advice they give to their students, as a record of the student's engagement with the supervisory team. If you should experience any difficulties or have any cause for complaint about your supervision, you should advise your Director of Studies at an early stage so that the issue can be addressed.

Dealing with supervision problems

Naturally, it can be anticipated that the relationship between the student and their supervisors is going to be a changing dynamic throughout the period of the research award – it's a long-term relationship! At least some subtle shifts in the power differentials can be expected as you grow in confidence, and most supervisors will have experienced some dramatic and challenging changes in the balance of their relationships with some students. Most reported difficulties have been attributed to mismatched prior expectations on each side of the supervisory relationship (Frame & Allen, 2002; Chiang, 2003). If any circumstances arise that might affect your ability to continue to progress with your studies you need to contact your Director of Studies at once, so that they can advise you on how to proceed. If you feel uncomfortable about discussing this with your own supervisors, then there will be a clearly designated system for accessing an independent member of staff who will act as a Personal Tutor within the department. There will also be an annual review system in place that gives all students an opportunity to raise any concerns they have regarding their supervision arrangements. Hopefully, your Director of Studies should not be surprised by any new issues raised at that point in the year. Out of an extensive listing of reasons for dissatisfaction cited by students, one outstanding issue appears to be a particularly high expectation for the supervisor's availability. This issue could be largely averted by initial agreements to establish preferred contact arrangements and timescales for keeping in touch. However, there will always be times when the student perceives an urgent need for feedback, to which one hopes the supervisors would try to respond as promptly as possible.

Successful completion of your research degree

All universities are now subject to increasingly high targets for timely completion of research degrees and consequently impose much stricter timescales on postgraduate research students. Each HEI will have provision for students to apply for additional time if needed on the grounds of illness or other genuine extenuating personal circumstances. But it would be much harder, for example, for a part-time student to make a case for leniency on the basis of pressure of work in their clinical post. This is why it is important to think about the advice at the start of this section before embarking on this path. Then once the project proposal has been agreed, you hope that your project will run smoothly and that you won't encounter any unexpected difficulties in participant recruitment or in the conduct of the study which will adversely affect your completion. For this reason, in the current climate of rapid organizational change, it can be advisable to plan to 'front-load' the data collection element of your research study: that is, to gather your research data as soon as possible once you have received the necessary ethical approvals, so that you will be less anxious about losing access to the participants and settings you need if local services are restructured. Your supervisory team will advise you on the most appropriate protocol for your study which may allow you to 'future-proof' your project in this way. Longitudinal studies will necessarily pose greater challenges in this regard, although your supervisory team will advise you on this. The university research office will also generally expect you to arrange a letter of 'support in principle' from the organization or stakeholders where you hope to recruit participants for your research, before they will agree for you to start your proposed project.

How can I get funding for my research?

Funding a research degree

The inescapable question when you apply to enrol at a university will be 'who is going to pay the fees'? The NHS Service Level Agreements mentioned above are unlikely to cover fees for research degrees, although it is always worthwhile asking whether your employer might be prepared to at least make a contribution to the enrolment fees. Before you start this conversation, be ready to list all the benefits to the team and to the wider organization that would result from their investment in building your research capability. Ensure you are familiar with the strategic research aims of the organization where you work, and show how your proposed project would contribute to that.

This section of the chapter offers advice about a range of possible funding sources, only some of which cover enrolment fees for a higher degree. The National Institute for Health Research (NIHR) Clinical Academic Training Programme was opened to Allied Health Professionals in 2009. This scheme comprised bursaries at Masters and Doctoral level for fully-funded studentships, including full payment of course fees and salary replacement costs to the NHS employer. Hopefully, there will continue to be similar opportunities in the future, but it must be anticipated that these places will be fiercely competitive. For this reason, it is recommended that you seek assistance from experienced colleagues and other contacts, as well as allowing yourself a significant length of time to prepare an application. Submissions hastily compiled over the last few days before the closing date are highly unlikely to be successful.

Internships and research posts

Another way to gain direct experience of working in a research environment is to look for opportunities to work as a Research Assistant on research projects or programmes that have already been funded. These contracts will always be fixed-term (often over one, two or three years), so it won't give you any long-term job security. Increasingly, there are also opportunities to work on Internships which often run for just a few weeks as part of a larger research project; although these are sometimes only open to undergraduate students over the summer vacation. Keeping in touch with your local HEI contacts will ensure you are aware of any such opportunities. Working as a contract researcher can offer an exciting opportunity to further develop your skills and widen your horizons within the research community. The Principal Researchers who are leading these teams will always be preparing bids for future projects, so there may be prospects for further research work. This can be a way for you to progressively build your own research CV of project experience and co-authored publications, aiming to be ready to be the lead applicant yourself in due course.

Funding a clinical research project

Getting ready to submit a bid for funding

As discussed in earlier chapters, it is recommended that you start to build your experience of active involvement in the research process through relatively small-scale projects within your own caseload and work setting, which have minimal resource cost implications. Hopefully, you will have support from your managers, colleagues and possibly even local students. In this way, you can start to build up collaborative working partnerships with colleagues who already have more experience of research, and together you will start to plan for what you could achieve if only you could secure some substantial funding for your next project. As you might imagine, there's increasingly tough competition for any available resources, but as long as you are realistic in your aspirations, you can make a start. Keep your focus firmly on the anticipated clinical application of your proposed project and start to reflect on the following pointers. The advice in this section cannot guarantee you success, but will help to steer you closer to your goal.

Any potential funder is going to want to be satisfied that your proposal is well-designed, relevant and timely. Importantly, they will also want to be assured that you have the necessary expertise and experience to carry out the project. Research sponsors will want to be satisfied that your proposed project will deliver the highest quality findings, whilst still representing good value for money. In your funding application you need to specify the journals or professional conferences where you plan to submit the findings of your proposed project, to demonstrate that you have already thought about the audiences who will recognize the relevance of your work. The costings need to be realistic and reasonable to match the deliverables in your application; don't be tempted to submit a guessed budget, as you could either lose the bid for an over-inflated proposal or, worse still, succeed and have to deliver a project with badly insufficient resourcing. These are some of the key reasons why bids are more often successful when the applicants already have a proven track record of project management. So when you are starting out as a researcher, you need to work alongside other more experienced teams whilst you build your own research CV. The following points are suggested as a useful checklist for planning how to start to set out your project budget, although of course many sponsors will specify very exacting requirements for this:

- Staff costs – Project Manager, Research Assistants, clerical support

- Treatment costs and materials

- Participants' travel expenses and refreshments

- Travel expenses and refreshments for Steering Group meetings

- Admin resources including printing, postage, etc.

- Dissemination costs including conference fees, on-line journal fee, etc.

The National Institute for Health Research (NIHR) exists to promote high-quality healthcare research across England, by funding and commissioning health and social care research. In 2008, the NIHR launched ten regional Research Design Service (RDS) centres, to provide expert support for staff working in the NHS in England to prepare research bids, particularly for submission to the main NIHR funding streams. The NIHR hosts a website (www.rdinfo. org.uk) that comprises a wealth of information about all aspects of healthcare research, including lists of research funding sources and sponsors. Many of these calls for research proposals are also open to healthcare professionals working across the rest of the UK and these sites are highly recommended as a resource to be bookmarked and checked regularly. There is also a link to this site from the RCSLT website members' area. Additionally, there are links on the RCSLT website to a wide number of research grants and bursaries that are directly relevant to SLT clinical practice; including awards for clinical service innovations.

Local funding sources

Many other much smaller organizations, including local charities, have also been receptive to applications for relatively modest SLT-related research bids and it is certainly well worth investigating a wide range of local groups such as Rotary Clubs. These sources have been particularly successful for projects that promote improved services for local groups, especially when there is resonance with key social issues or priority themes. However, it is essential to thoroughly familiarize yourself with the strategic priorities of any organizations prior to starting to draft your application and before making an approach to them. The best advice is to consider potential funding sources very early, so that you can tailor your project proposal to match the key priorities of the sponsor you've identified. It can also be vitally important to your research CV to show that you have successfully secured a number of small bids before you aim for more substantive funds.

National funding streams

Sources of funding for healthcare research in the UK are increasingly competitive, but nonetheless Allied Health Professionals have every opportunity to bid for these monies.

National funding streams increasingly expect that research proposals demonstrate each of the following elements: innovation, impact, interdisciplinarity and internationalization. NIHR research streams additionally include calls for project proposals from NHS staff with the aim of achieving flexibility and sustainability for future service delivery. Over recent years, healthcare research sponsors also increasingly expect to see evidence of active patient or service-user involvement (PPI) in the development as well as the conduct of the project. It is worthwhile seeking out opportunities to attend workshops on participatory research, or finding colleagues who already have some experience of involving service users in research. The INVOLVE national advisory group website also provides valuable information and updates about supporting greater public involvement in health and social care research. The site also incorporates a database of projects, listing their funding sources as well as the research approaches used.

Over recent decades, funding for much mainstream healthcare research in the UK has come from the national funding councils; particularly from the Medical Research Council – MRC (www.mrc.ac.uk) and the Economic and Social Research Council – ESRC (www.esrc.ac.uk). The Research Councils all provide a range of funding opportunities, including competition calls, open grants and fellowship schemes. Innovative clinical research projects are welcomed, but the Councils generally expect applications from teams that include experienced researchers rather than novice researchers alone. There are also a number of other large organizations, including charitable bodies, that are noted for sponsoring research relevant to aspects of SLT professional practice. The following list includes some examples but is by no means exhaustive:

Action Medical Research (www.action.org)

Cancer Research UK (www.cancerresearchuk.org)

Leverhulme Trust (www.leverhulme.ac.uk)

Nuffield Foundation (www.nuffieldfoundation.org)

Stroke Association (www.stroke.org.uk)

Wellcome Trust (www.wellcome.ac.uk)

An additional useful strategy is to regularly check the GRANTfinder service (www.grantfinder.co.uk), which offers access to a fully searchable database of research funders across the UK. The full service requires a subscription and it's possible that your employer, or one of your collaborators, may already have access to this service. There are also free options that are more limited, but can still be very useful, including GRANTnet (www.grantnet.com).

Getting support for research in the workplace

Support from managers

It is essential that your managers know how serious you are about becoming research-active: you certainly do not want to miss out on any opportunities for research-related experiences simply because they weren't aware that you would have been interested. So you need to make sure you discuss this in your annual appraisals, which will additionally support any requests you make for skills development and training needs. Your managers are increasingly responsible for demonstrating that the clinical service provides good value for money, as well as measurable clinical outcomes. Your SLT service is likely to have a wide range of exemplars of exciting and innovative practice that have been developed by experienced therapists, including you. However, without any supporting evidence of effectiveness, the sustainability of this good practice can be under threat as services are rationalized and restructured. Offering to help design, analyze and report service evaluations can be a very good way to show how you can apply your critical thinking skills, as well as your systematic approach to undertaking a project. It also gives you an opportunity to discuss with the managers your ideas for well-designed research projects that you could feasibly undertake within your own clinical caseload and routine practice, which will further contribute to the professional evidence base.

Support from colleagues

Research methods have been described in detail earlier in this book and there are also many clear introductory texts and guides to research approaches (see recommendations for Further Reading at the end of this chapter). For the clinical projects you plan to undertake, you will probably need to demonstrate increased credibility of your findings; for example by showing that the clinical assessments were undertaken by someone other than the therapist who delivered intervention (blinding of assessors). If you work in a team of therapists, your greatest asset could be your own colleagues; who would be only too happy to assist you in this way even if they are not ready to see themselves as taking the lead in research activities. There are many other ways too in which your colleagues might be able to help to support your research projects: from giving feedback on your draft proposals, contributing to expert consensus gathering, and recruiting patient/client participants. And when you reach the stage of preparing to present the findings of your research study, your colleagues could also give you valuable constructive feedback. You will, of course, need to be mindful of following the agreed participant recruitment protocol and the good practice principles of confidentiality and anonymity when you discuss your projects with colleagues. But nevertheless, they will be able to give you the most invaluable reality check that your research question and results are meaningful and valid and have potential applications in a clinical context.

Support from R&D Officers

If you work in an NHS organization, it is highly recommended that you build a good relationship with the Research and Development (R&D) officers. Their principal role is in research governance, so you will need their support for any projects that you want to undertake within the workplace. In the first instance, they will be able to give you their advice about whether your proposal constitutes audit, service evaluation or research – which can very often be a grey area. Research proposals will require ethical approval from the NHS Research Ethics Service (NRES) as well as local R&D governance approval. In some organizations, the R&D officers offer a range of training in research skills and update sessions that are open to all staff. They may also offer you assistance in completing the NHS on-line application for ethics approval (IRAS), which will be extremely welcome as this can seem a very daunting prospect the first time you encounter it.

The R&D officers have responsibility for monitoring all research activity for the local patient population, which will mostly comprise engagement in large drugs trials, recruitment to portfolio studies, etc. You might get the impression that they are less interested in supporting your small-scale projects or assisting you to secure funding or other resources to continue to be research-active. However, you should persist in letting them know your research interests and aspirations. Ask about the organization's strategic aims for building research capacity and capability and emphasize how your research work has the potential to impact on quality standards and the patient experience of local services.

Professional networks

Chapter 1 discussed the RCSLT's Research Strategy, launched in 2009. More recently, the national network of RCSLT clinical Specific Interest Groups (SIGs) have been encouraged to work to actively support and operationalize this research agenda, as part of providing high-quality continuing professional development. RCSLT worked with a number of SLT researchers and clinicians to produce a range of critical appraisal activities that SIGs can use to focus on the relevant evidence base. Through this structured approach to reviewing the existing evidence, it is hoped that the group members will become better equipped to generate new research in their own area of practice.

There are also many benefits to actively networking with other research-active healthcare professionals. In 2011, the Allied Health Professions Research

Network (AHPRN) was launched across the UK. This is a network of more than 20 cross-professional research interest groups, based on a hub infrastructure previously supported by the Chartered Society of Physiotherapy (CSP) and is also supported by the Research Forum for Allied Health Professionals (RFAHP). Two pilot hubs led this initiative, although it is expected that each group will function differently in response to local issues. For example, one of the pilot sites, which is co-hosted by the University of Central Lancashire and the University of Cumbria, has focused on delivering a rolling programme of "Masterclass" workshops in research skills. These sessions provide training opportunities for therapists who are completely new to research, as well as refreshers for others who already have some experience; everyone is welcome. The AHPRN groups also offer a supportive forum for therapists to discuss their ideas for research projects and to exchange advice about funding sources. Group members have the opportunity to present recently completed work, with an emphasis on their research approach and their experiences of the research process, as well as their topic and findings. Subsidised by the AHPRN funding, a number of clinicians have been supported to undertake small-scale clinical research projects, and to submit their findings for publication.

The AHPRN groups are open to all clinicians, wherever they are working. For therapists working in the NHS, there are also research networks hosted by some of the Strategic Health Authority AHP leads. As the NHS restructures continue, it is more important than ever to establish contact with research-active colleagues from a range of clinical backgrounds, and to keep in touch with each other for future potential collaborations and mutual exchange of helpful advice.

Collaborative links between clinical services and universities

You don't need to be enrolled for a research award to take advantage of working closely with relevant contacts in local HEIs. Many NHS organizations host research interest groups which provide an opportunity for clinicians to make contact with each other, as well as with more experienced academic research colleagues. There are also often regular research seminars, where research staff and postgraduate research students present their current work. These seminars are open to all interested local clinical practitioners, and are often held at the end of the working day so that it is easier for everyone to attend. These sessions are invaluable opportunities for keeping updated about other on-going research projects, as well as for comparing experiences about sources of research funding. Making links with other research-active colleagues at these events can lead to opportunities for putting together collaborative research bids. Joint bids between clinical services and academic teams are a requirement for many funding streams in healthcare research, so local HEIs will be very interested indeed in exploring opportunities to work with you.

Virtual research networks

Many HEIs have their own web-based forums and on-line research communities, which may be useful to investigate. These could be useful for identifying links across highly subject-specific or specialist clinical groups, in line with specified research topics. There are also a number of broader postgraduate networks which give an effective overview of the most current and salient research in related fields, as well as potentially valuable links with key researchers. An example of the type of useful web-based sources within health is the RDLearning site (http://www.rdlearning.org.uk) hosted by the University of Leeds, which is an invaluable reference for a very wide range of research training opportunities and news. Another particularly valuable site relevant to health and social care is the Contact Help Advice and Information Network – CHAIN (http://chain. ulcc.ac.uk/chain/index.html), which provides a forum for multiprofessional and cross-agency networking and the dissemination of research news.

Taking the next step as a research-active clinician

The over-arching theme of this book has been about clinically-driven research. As a therapist, your priorities and passions have always been focused on providing the highest quality care for the people you work with – your patients and clients. Wanting to answer the question of how you can optimize the outcomes for the people who use our services, as well as improving the way you and your colleagues deliver these services, is the fundamental basis of applied clinical research. Chapters 4 to 8 have shone the spotlight on the range of drivers for research questions about the perceptions of service users as well as using standardized clinical outcome measures. When you reflect on your own clinical practice, certainly at least one of these themes will have resonated with the issues that you keep turning over in your mind – the concerns that drive us all. As a clinician, you draw upon your own experiences as well as those of the people you work with every day, to underpin your decision-making. So, the very first check to answer the question *"How can I be sure I have found the right research question?"* relates to the purpose of your research idea. If you can explain how answering this question is going to help you in your clinical practice, then it passes the *"so what"* test. The first three chapters also reinforce the message that, as experienced clinicians, it is important that we recognize that we are optimally placed to contribute to the collective evidence base for our profession.

Once you have identified a specific relevant question, you will be able to start to consider how that can be answered. Chapter 2 introduced a framework for developing a research protocol and emphasized how the methodology in the research design needs to match the research question. Practice-based evidence can comprise a range of research designs, as illustrated in the preceding chapters in Part II. Providing that these studies are well-designed, even very small-scale projects that you can undertake within your existing caseload (and without the need for any external funding) could be one of the most realistic and achievable ways to get started as a researcher. Engaging in a small-scale study in this way will help you to gain invaluable first-hand experience of all stages of the research process. However, it is strongly recommended that you take the chance to benefit from the support of more experienced colleagues, as has been discussed in this chapter. You will be able to make a genuine contribution to the collective professional evidence base, providing that you disseminate your findings, as Rosemarie has encouraged us to do in Chapter 9.

You will now be nearly ready to take the plunge into the next stage of your research-active career. The sections in this chapter have signposted a range of training and skills-development options, to boost your potential for success in planning and undertaking practice-based research. The discussions above have also given you an insight into the fierce competition for research funding; you will certainly need to be tenacious and patient. But do stay optimistic – and be opportunistic. Seize every chance to make contacts across clinical and academic environments with other individuals who may be able to assist you on your research journey.

References

Anderson, L. W. & Krathwohl, D. (Eds) (2001) *A Taxonomy for Learning, Teaching and Assessing: A Revision of Bloom's Taxonomy of Educational Objectives*. London: Longman.

Baxter Magolda, M. (1996) Epistemological development in graduate and professional education. *Review of Higher Education* **19(3)**, 283–304.

Bloom, B. S. (Ed.) (1956) *Taxonomy of Educational Objectives: The Classification of Educational Goals*. London: Longman.

Chiang, K-H. (2003) Learning experiences of doctoral students in UK universities. *International Journal of Sociology and Social Policy* **3** (2/3), 4–32.

Frame, I. A. & Allen, L. (2002) A flexible approach to PhD research training. *Quality Assurance in Education* **12** (2), 98–103.

Lewis, V. & Habeshaw, S. (1997) *53 Interesting Ways to Supervise Student Projects, Dissertations and Theses*. Bristol: Technical and Educational Services Ltd.

Schon, D. (1983) *The Reflective Practitioner*. London: Basic Books

van der Gaag, A. & Anderson, C. (2005) The geography of professional practice: Swamps and icebergs. In: C. Anderson, & A. van der Gaag (Eds) *Speech and Language Therapy: Issues in Professional Practice*. London: Whurr.

Further reading

Fish, D. & Coles, C. (1998) *Developing Professional Judgement in Healthcare. Learning Through the Critical Appreciation of Practice*. London: Butterworth Heinemann.

Hickson, M. (2008) *Research Handbook for Health Care Professionals*. Chichester: Wiley-Blackwell.

Moore, A. P. & Lyon, P. (Eds) (2009) *Getting Involved in Research: A Pocket Guide*. London: National Physiotherapy Research Network.

Pring, T. (2004) *Research Methods in Communication Disorders*. London: Whurr.

Resources

Ethics approval for research:

Integrated Research Application System (IRAS) https://www.myresearchproject.org.uk

National Research Ethics Service http://www.nres.npsa.nhs.uk

Funding for research:

National Institute for Health Research www.nihr.ac.uk

Patient/service-user involvement in research

INVOLVE national advisory network www.invo.org.uk

Research information and news updates;

Allied Health Professions Research Network http://tinyurl.com/cpxkjgu

Contact Help and Advice Information network http://chain.ulcc.ac.uk/chain/index.html

Research and development information www.rdinfo.org.uk

RCSLT Special Interest Groups (SIGs) http://www.rcslt.org/members/sigs/intro

Royal College of Speech and Language Therapists www.rcslt.org

Research training:

RD Learning http://www.rdlearning.org.uk

Quality Assurance Agency Code of Practice for standards for registration of postgraduate students www.qaa.ac.uk/academicinfrastructure/codeofpractice/section1/defult.asp

UK Research Councils Best Practice guidelines for postgraduate training

www.epsrc.ac.uk/PostgraduateTraining/JointStatementOnSkillsTraining.htm

11 Summary

Corinne Dobinson and Yvonne Wren

As you read this final chapter, we hope that you will feel equipped and ready to start on your journey towards gathering practice-based evidence. Questions that have puzzled you as a clinician can now be considered in a meaningful and systematic way, consistent with the processes and requirements inherent within NHS research systems.

While it is a requirement that our clinical practice is driven by the evidence base, the evidence base should, of course, also reflect the concerns of clinicians and inform the decisions we make in our everyday work. As clinicians, we are ideally placed to generate research questions that are directly relevant to the interface between services, clients and commissioners. Our broader question could be inspired by formal reflection on our clinical practice or by a throw-away comment made by a client as they leave the clinic. Indeed, our regular contact with service users allows us to involve them at every stage of evidence gathering. Practised-based evidence is the gathering of evidence within the context of everyday clinical work. Resources for evidence gathering in the workplace can be limited, but it is still an activity that can be engaged in by those of us who are prepared to spend a little time thinking and planning methodically.

The steps described in all the chapters and illustrated in Chapter 2 will help us with this; the authors remind us, however, that although these have an order, they do not necessarily progress in a linear fashion, but more iteratively. This is exemplified particularly in the first stages where our broader clinical query becomes increasingly refined as we appraise the literature. The literature not only enables us to see what questions have already been answered and the level of evidence that already exists around the subject, but also what approaches have been used to answer similar questions. We can target the most relevant papers by using search terms based on the key words from our broader question. When searching for studies that provide efficacy outcomes, useful literature will be meta-analyses and systematic reviews; here, strict inclusion criteria are used to assess the quality of the work conducted so far and to appraise the value of their outcomes or to combine them by using special methods of analysis. If we are searching for literature about processes, however, for example training approaches or methods for gathering views, we might wish to broaden our search to include areas beyond our clinical field or even outside of speech and language therapy. Our hospital library service can be an excellent source of support both in conducting literature searches for us or by providing us with training in how to do this.

By refining our broader question to one that is specific and manageable, we are better able to consider how we might answer it. We will be increasingly specific about *who, what* and *how* we will investigate. Our inclusion and exclusion criteria, in relation to our sample, will be based on a rational argument informed by our literature review and clinical experience; yet we must be careful also that they aren't so stringent that we have difficulty recruiting enough participants or including sufficient data. Our methods may be qualitative or quantitative, or include both to answer a question from different perspectives. Our design and analysis will be determined by these decisions and also influenced by the resources and time available to us. Once we have a specific question, it makes it easier for us to seek support from others who have more expertise in research design and analysis.

If we are measuring the outcome of a specific intervention, the intervention and the way in which it is delivered will need to be consistent. This will be more achievable if we have manualized it. We will need to define and rationalize what we consider to be a 'difference', if this is what we aim to measure. Our outcome measures need to be valid, so we know they capture data that are relevant to the question we are asking. They will also need to be reliable and not be subject to bias. This is the case whether we are looking at very specific changes in impairment or capturing the broader effects of the intervention on activity and participation or quality of life. With respect to these broader measures, we also need to consider whether we will run the risk of introducing bias should we use proxy data collection rather than self-report and whether or not it might be feasible to use both.

When seeking the views of others, perhaps to improve services or to see how feasible and acceptable a novel intervention is, we might wish to capture a broad and rich data set that is unrestricted by the specificity of a particular measure. Focus groups and interviews provide us with this opportunity. We are reminded, though, that when gathering the views of people who have communication difficulty, we need to plan in advance how we will present the subject matter and have flexible means of gathering their feedback. We must also consider this when feeding back the results of a study to those who were involved.

As clinicians and managers we hold the key to a vast amount of information. Gathering data on our existing caseload can help us see if our service is fit for purpose, adheres to the evidence base and meets the wishes of funding bodies and the population. It can also help us to see how it might need to develop in the future. We might undertake a retrospective data collection from existing sources, if we have the correct information at hand; alternatively, we might start to collect data prospectively, organizing this in such a way that we acquire relevant information to answer our question, or those asked by others. We must be cautious that we identify and discriminate between the exact information we are asked to report on and that which we don't need.

Our service-users and their families are a rich source of information and we will need to ensure we are including their views and opinions when service planning. Their experiences will also be crucial when developing and evaluating new approaches to therapy. When designing and conducting a research project, our clients and the public can be involved at each stage of the process. They may be the source of research questions, can help us design information sheets and other materials appropriate for our target population, and can help us in the dissemination of our findings.

When we derive findings from a piece of work that is well thought out and executed, it is our responsibility to act upon them accordingly. Ultimately, if appropriate, this could lead to a change of practice or service delivery, but we should also disseminate them to those who might benefit from them. When we are starting out in gathering evidence, especially when our project is small, we can forget how much we have progressed and it is easy to have a distorted view that no-one will be interested in what we have found; however, we will, more often than not, be pleasantly surprised at the interest people take and the questions people ask when we present our work. Being always mindful of the work's limitations, we need to identify our target audience and consider the best ways of reaching it. We need to think about the most appropriate medium through which to present our findings, and pitch the tone and style in a way that best communicates our message by giving consideration to our target audience. By writing up as we go along, and keeping a project journal, we will ease the process of dissemination by being familiar and confident about our evidence and its limitations.

Gathering evidence can seem a daunting task if we don't have the right skills, or lack confidence in those we do have, but we must remember that others are usually willing to help and support us. The support we seek will come from different sources; from trusted 'mates' with whom we can discuss and re-discuss our potential question and ideas, to that offered by our own organization and other institutions. The advice of people who have more experience than us will be invaluable and we will feel more confident if we approach them with questions we have thought through beforehand. In addition to developing a network of support, we might wish to form collaborations with others, to pool our resources and approach a question collectively; possibly applying for joint funding to support costs.

Our motivation for gathering evidence could be to simply find an answer to a question that has been bugging us in our clinical work; on the other hand, we could have more personal aspirations for conducting a project, such as gaining a higher degree. If so, we need to consider what type of degree is right for us and which institution might provide the right support and supervision. We need to investigate what funding opportunities might be open to us and consider how studying for a degree will fit in with our work and home life. Talking to others who have been through this experience can be helpful to us in making those decisions. We will also need to reflect what skills we might need to acquire and what training is available. While we are studying for our degree, making links with others who are research active will be a good source of support, enabling us to share our experiences and get research news and updates.

Whatever our motivation to gather evidence, we will feel more confident in our findings if we have approached our specific question with a clear understanding of the necessary processes involved in answering it and how to carry them out. Whether our findings turn out to agree with our predicted outcome or are in fact a complete surprise, we will also be aware of their limitations. We may be content with them as they are or, more often than not, they will stimulate our curiosity, generating further questions or the wish to establish a more robust answer. With the tools and knowledge you have gained through reading this book, the only thing left to do is start your research project, confident that the knowledge that is acquired through your activity will help to increase the evidence base for speech and language therapy and, ultimately, improve outcomes for the clients we seek to serve.

Glossary

A priori This means that you have developed a theory or a hypothesis at the start of your investigation (or analysis) that informs subsequent steps. For example, you have an a priori hypothesis that you wish to test; it suggests that you already have a set of assumptions that you wish to find out about. Of course, even if we don't have an explicit a priori theory, we often have a set of assumptions that can impact on how we conduct research. Trying to be clear about our own assumptions at the start of a project is a useful way of surfacing our own bias.

Analytic or Theoretical codes To go beyond description and start to categorize and analyze the data.

Bias The process or consequence of systematic errors or inaccuracies in the design and/or conduct of research that influences the findings and therefore leads to an inaccurate result.

Central tendency The 'average'; which can be described as the mean, mode or median.

Clinimetric An approach to developing quality of life scales that uses groups of individuals, with a relevant clinical condition, to rate and then select potential question items.

Confidence interval (CI) An indication of the margin of error where a p value has been obtained. The greater the interval, the less certain one is of the true value of p.

Critical appraisal The objective evaluation of research papers.

Database An electronic catalogue of research publications (in journals).

Dependent variable (DV) In experimental research, the variable in which you wish to measure an effect (for example, sound pressure level, number of items correctly named, etc.).

Descriptive codes These provide a summary description of what is in the transcript or text. Codes can be based upon Themes, Topics, Ideas, Concepts, Terms, Phrases or Keywords.

Descriptive statistics	A description of what data look like.
Dissemination plan	A documented strategy for sharing the knowledge gained from a project.
Feasibility study	A small-scale study which tests out procedures, materials, outcome measures, recruitment rates and logistical issues in preparation for a larger study.
Five-phase model for clinical-outcome research	A model that provides an organizational structure for the systematic investigation of the effects of an intervention or treatment (see Robey, 2004).
Focus group	An informal meeting to discuss people's views and ideas about a specific topic, problem or experience.
Gantt chart	A visual representation of a research project timetable with all tasks listed against their time allocation.
Hawthorn effect	Change in the independent variable (IV) which can be brought about by participants simply having attention paid to them.
Hypothesis	A prediction of the expected outcome of your research question.
Inclusion and exclusion criteria	The criteria upon which participants are recruited into a study.
Independent variable (IV)	In experimental research, the variable that you manipulate to introduce an effect (on the dependent variable).
In-depth interviews	These aim to explore the deeper meanings and feelings associated with the area of investigation.
Interlibrary loans	The process by which a library will obtain a publication that is not in their collection. They usually come from the British Library and there is a small charge.
Internal consistency	The extent to which different versions of an assessment match in their reliability to test the same thing.

Interquartile range (IQR)	The range of data held in the middle 50% of the values.
IRAS	Integrated Research Approval Service – gives information and access to the process of UK ethical and R&D approval.
Iterative	In a research context, this usually means that a particular cycle of the data collection and/or analysis is being repeated and that data or findings from the first cycle or stage will inform or impact in some way upon subsequent stages.
Likert Scale	A method of scaling responses to questionnaire items that enables the researcher to rank individuals' responses.
Margin of error	The difference in scores on a test that you would obtain if you repeated it under equivalent conditions; that is, with the same participants, judges, same time of day, etc.
Meta-analysis	A statistical technique for combining the results of separate smaller studies to be equivalent to one larger scale investigation.
Null hypothesis	When it is expected that there will be no change associated with the independent variable.
One-tailed (or directional)	When an outcome is predicted to go in a particular direction (i.e., either positive or negative).
Open access	Full versions of online journal articles that are available free to the public.
Operational definitions	Specification of variables and processes involved in an experiment.
Patient and Public Involvement (PPI)	The active involvement of patient and public views in healthcare services and the evaluation of them.
Placebo condition	An intervention that should not influence the variables you wish to change.
Probability	An estimation of the outcomes occurring by chance; usually represented as p. A p value smaller than 5% (0.005) is

considered to be statistically significant. *P* is an approximation of probability and so is usually accompanied by the confidence interval.

Protocol   The document specifying all procedures to be carried out in a research study.

Psychometric   An approach to developing quality of life scales that uses statistical modelling to select potential question items and validate them on a representative sample of a population.

Pygmalion effect   Change in the independent variable (IV) brought about by the power of expectation on behalf of the participant or the researcher.

Qualitative   A research methodology that seeks to provide a deep understanding of human experience, which is underpinned by a subjective philosophy throughout the process of research design, data collection, analysis and reporting.

Quality of life (QoL)   A person's perception of their social, psychological and physical health.

Quantitative   A research methodology based around the quantification of empirical data. Unlike qualitative research, quantitative research is founded on principles of objectivity and often includes hypothesis testing.

Range   The lowest to the highest value obtained .

Reference Manager   Software to organize references and citations; a real time saver!

Reliability   The extent to which results are consistent if an assessment is repeated over time (test re-test reliability), with different raters (inter-rater reliability), or the same person rescoring the same data on a separate occasion (intra-rater reliability).

Sampling   The process a researcher takes when selecting a smaller group of participants from a (clinical) population.

Search terms   The words entered into a database to find specified literature.

Stakeholder	An individual, group or organization with some level of interest in your treatment or service.
Standard deviation	A figure representing the spread of data around the mean.
Systematic review	A review of published research relating to a specified question; studies are systematically appraised with reference to the methods used, how they were conducted and the validity and reliability of the outcomes.
Two-tailed (or non-directional)	When the direction of the outcome is not predicted (i.e., not sure if it will be positive or negative).
Validity	The extent to which the chosen assessment is a true measure of the variables selected for measurement.

Index